Books should be returned to the SDH Library on or before
the date stamped above unless a renewal has been arranged

Salisbury District Hospital Library

Telephone: Salisbury (01722) 336262 extn. 4432 / 33

Out of hours answer machine in operation

Developing Online Learning Environments in Nursing Education

Carol A. O'Neil, RN, CNE, PhD, is an Assistant Professor at the University of Maryland School of Nursing. She is Codirector of the Institute for Educators in Nursing and Health Professions and Director of the RN to BSN/MS program. Dr. O'Neil is a Web Initiative in Teaching (WIT) Fellow. She has journal articles about teaching and learning online and has presented her research and experiences at both international and national conferences.

Cheryl A. Fisher, RN, EdD, is the Program Manager for Professional Development at the National Institutes of Health Clinical Center in Bethesda, Maryland. She received her doctorate in instructional technology from Towson University and has a postgraduate certificate in nursing informatics and in nursing education. She is responsible for all the central education at the NIH Clinical Center and is actively working to reconceptualize the courses utilizing technology. She is as an adjunct professor for the University of Maryland and teaches graduate courses in nursing informatics.

Susan K. Newbold, RN-BC, PhD, FAAN, FHIMSS, is an Associate Professor of Nursing Informatics at Vanderbilt School of Nursing. She has taught online courses since 1999 for three schools of nursing. Susan is certified in Nursing Informatics by the American Nurses Credentialing Center, a Fellow of the American Academy of Nursing and a Fellow of the Health Care Management and Systems Society. Dr. Newbold has made many presentations on health care informatics in the United States and internationally. She is the cofounder of CARING, a national nursing informatics special interest group. Dr. Newbold has numerous publications to her credit including coediting three editions of *Nursing Informatics: Where Caring and Technology Meet.*

Developing Online Learning Environments in Nursing Education

SECOND EDITION

CAROL A. O'NEIL, RN, CNE, PhD

CHERYL A. FISHER, RN, EdD

SUSAN K. NEWBOLD, RN-BC, PhD, FAAN, FHIMSS

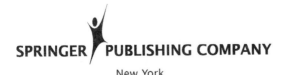

SPRINGER PUBLISHING COMPANY

New York

Springer Publishing Company, LLC
11 West 42nd Street
New York, NY 10036
www.springerpub.com

Acquisitions Editor: Allan Graubard
Production Manager: Kelly J. Applegate
Cover design: Mimi Flow
Composition: Publication Services, Inc.

09 10 11/ 5 4 3

Library of Congress Cataloging-in-Publication Data

O'Neil, Carol A.
    Developing online learning environments in nursing education / Carol A. O'Neil, Cheryl A. Fisher, Susan K. Newbold. — 2nd ed.
        p. ; cm.
    Rev. ed. of: Developing an online course / Carol A. O'Neil, Cheryl A. Fisher, Susan K. Newbold. c2004.
    Includes bibliographical references and index.
    ISBN 978-0-8261-6902-0 (hardcover)
    1. Nursing—Study and teaching.   2. Internet in education.   I. Fisher, Cheryl A.   II. Newbold, Susan K.   III. Newbold, Susan K. Developing an online course.   IV. Title.
    [DNLM: 1. Education, Nursing—methods.   2. Curriculum.   3. Education, Distance.   4. Internet. WY 18 O58d 2008]
    RT73.O59 2008
    610.73071'1—dc22

                                                                            2008028440

Printed in the United States of America by Bang Printing

We dedicate this book to our families
for their tolerance and patience
through this second edition.

Contents

Preface   xi

Chapter 1   Introduction to Teaching and Learning
with Technology   1
Carol A. O'Neil

Chapter 2   Pedagogy Associated with Learning
in Online Environments   17
Carol A. O'Neil

Chapter 3   Infrastructure Considerations for
Online Learning: Student, Faculty,
and Technical Support   35
Cheryl A. Fisher

Chapter 4   Technologies and Competencies Needed for
Online Learning   57
Susan K. Newbold and Cheryl A. Fisher

Chapter 5   Reconceptualizing the Online Course   67
Carol A. O'Neil

Chapter 6   Designing the Online Learning Environment   83
                  Carol A. O'Neil

Chapter 7   Interacting and Communicating Online   99
                  Cheryl A. Fisher

Chapter 8   Course Management Methods   111
                  Cheryl A. Fisher

Chapter 9   Assessment and Evaluation of
                  Online Learning   135
                  Carol A. O'Neil and Cheryl A. Fisher

Chapter 10   Distance and Continuing Medical Education   151
                  William A. Sadera and Cheryl A. Fisher

Chapter 11   Using Technology in Teaching   167
                  Carol A. O'Neil

Chapter 12   Educating Patients for Positive Behavior
                  Change and Health Outcomes   179
                  Barbara Covington and Carol A. O'Neil

                  Index   193

Contributors

Barbara Covington, RN, PhD, possesses over 35 years experience in civilian and military health care systems and higher education, clinical simulation, distance education and health care informatics. During the past fifteen years, her consulting, teaching, publishing, and research has focused on academic infrastructure development and sustainment, including clinical simulation labs, using technology in clinical and academic settings, clinical simulation research and Nursing education, and health care systems low- to high-fidelity technology implementation across the United States and overseas. Her publications include books and journal articles focused on clinical simulation.

William A. Sadera, PhD, is an Associate Professor at Towson University, Towson, Maryland. Dr. Sadera currently serves as the Director of the Doctoral Program in Instructional Technology in Towson University's College of Education. He has been active in the field of Instructional Technology and Online Learning, having taught courses and conducted research on this topic for over ten years; his current research focuses on online professional development, pedagogy, and effective design.

Preface

In 1958 DARPA (Defense Advanced Research Projects Agency) developed a mechanism to communicate research data and Department of Defense (DOD) project information. This mechanism was the Web. Now celebrating 50 years in existence, the Web has grown from a means of communicating research to an integral part of our daily lives. The primary uses of the Web are for commerce, entertainment, and education.

In the past decade, the Web has impacted the way nurses teach students, teach patients, and provide continuing professional development. With the increasing availability of broadband and high-speed Internet, and increasing services and products from Internet service providers (ISPs), additional products for enhanced information and communication will continue to expand.

Web sites such as Web-MD (Webmd.com), which advertises that it has over 16 million users every month, provides information about health to the public. Online "Ask-a-Nurse" sites are available for the public to get answers to specific questions about health (www.msha.com/body.cfm?id=26). These sites continue to increase in numbers as increasing quantities of health information become available and as consumers of health information become increasingly more computer literate.

Hospitals and health care providers depend on internal networks and Web sites (intranets) for training employees and providing educational requirements for staff. Certifications are becoming fully or partially provided on the Web by continuing education departments, private continuing education companies, and other vendors.

The traditional "go-somewhere-where-the-weather-is-beautiful-and-the-sun-is-shining" three-day conference is moving online. Conference presentations and meetings are now taking place in the form of "Webinars," thereby providing a speaker and a presentation without having to physically be together.

Technology has also changed the way we teach. Research has repeatedly shown that learning can take place as effectively online as it does in traditional face-to-face learning environments. Because of these trends, we have added three new chapters to this second edition. We expanded the focus from teaching the nursing student to the consumer and the working adult professional. Additionally, we added a chapter dedicated to teaching with technology.

The focus of this book is for nurses who are developing online health education and information for health consumers and professional peers and students. This may include:

- developing online courses in nursing education;
- developing health education information;
- developing training or certification programs to enhance knowledge or skills.

This book is about using. It is about using the Web to teach student nurses, to train or retrain nurses, to certify competencies and skills, and to communicate. The nurse performing these activities needs a set of knowledge and skills such as pedagogy, the study of learning and specifically learning through a guided constructivist model (Chapter 2); the infrastructure needed to facilitate online strategies (Chapter 3); the technology courseware and software needed to teach and communicate in online environments (Chapter 4); reconceptualizing learning material from face-to-face to online environments (Chapter 5); designing online learning environments (Chapter 6); communicating and interacting online (Chapter 7); managing online learning (Chapter 8); assessing and evaluating learning in online environments (Chapter 9); continuing education (Chapter 10); using technology in teaching (Chapter 11); and educating patients using technology (Chapter 12).

This book is about using the Web to impart information and to communicate. Therefore, teaching and learning in online environments is its focus.

Carol A. O'Neil
Cheryl A. Fisher

Introduction to Teaching and Learning with Technology

CAROL A. O'NEIL

1

Technology can be used for enhancing teaching in the classroom and for educating learners outside of the traditional classroom. When the learner and teacher are in the classroom, some examples of technologies that enhance teaching are "clickers," audience response systems (Martyn, 2007) in the classroom and simulation in the lab (Simulation Labs, 2004). When the learner and the teacher are separated by geography and time, the learning is called "distance learning" (Williams, Paprock, Covington, 1999). The Instructional Technology Council (n.d.) defines distance education as "the process of extending learning, or delivering instructional resource-sharing opportunities, to locations away from a classroom, building or site, to another classroom, building or site by using video, audio, computer, multimedia communications, or some combination of these with other traditional delivery methods."

The Internet can be accessed to create, teach, and learn in online learning environments. Online learning environments reduce time and space barriers to learning and thus are called "anytime, anywhere learning." Online learning environments can be totally online or can be partially online in hybrid or blended learning environments.

A hybrid learning experience includes both face-to-face learning as well as virtual or distance learning strategies.

Online learning is instructor moderated, instructor taught, instructor mentored, yet student self-directed. An online learning environment can comprise large discussion groups, small group discussions, individual activities, group activities, and various levels of interaction between and among students, faculty, and mentors. Material can be presented in a variety of ways, including videotaping, audio taping, films, links to Web sites that host online learning environments, charts, graphs, statistical data, formulas, and case studies. Interaction can be synchronous (real time) or asynchronous (delayed). Synchronous interaction means having a discussion by typing instead of talking, such as a chat room. Asynchronous communication entails leaving messages at a specific posting site that others in the learning environment can read at their convenience. Individual courses, groups of courses, and entire programs are offered online. The degree of Internet usage in a course can range from supplementing classroom learning to courses and programs that are offered completely online.

Online learners can attend traditional universities, such as Pennsylvania State University (www.worldcampus.psu.edu), or virtual universities, such as California Virtual University (www.california.edu or www.cvc.edu). In addition to online courses and programs, online journals focus on teaching and learning in online environments, such as the *Journal of Asynchronous Learning Networks* (www.sloan-c.org/publications/jaln/). There are also professional organizations that provide resources for online teaching and learning such as Educause (www.educause.edu) and Sloan-C (www.sloan-c.org).

HISTORICAL PERSPECTIVE OF TEACHING WITH TECHNOLOGY

Teaching at a distance is not new to education. There have been paper-based distance curricula in which learners enrolled in universities and received their learning packages in the mail. Early correspondence courses enabled learners and instructors to interact, although with a significant time lag between message production and reception (Woods & Baker, 2004). Television provided a medium for teaching and learning at a distance. Students in remote areas could use the television to obtain learning content. In the late 1960s, Schramm (1962) conducted studies which compared instructional television (ITV) with classroom instruction and summarized the results of more than 400 empirical studies. The findings of his research were that there is no significant difference between learning from a television or from a classroom.

As distance education progressed from correspondence courses to online learning, opportunities for interpersonal interaction also increased. Videoconferencing made it possible for learners and faculty to interact in real time. With the emergence of the Internet, particularly e-mail and the World Wide Web, it became possible to promote high degrees of interaction utilizing mainstream technology and cost-effective learning environments. The Center for Adult Learning purports that:

> Developments in technology and communications have brought about dramatic changes in both the learning needs and the way learning opportunities are delivered in business, labor, government, and academia. We are becoming a society in which continuous learning is central to effective participation as citizens and wage earners. Telecommunications technologies are not only transforming our needs for education and training, but they are expanding our capacity to respond to these needs. Distance learning, with a long history of serving isolated and remote learners, has now emerged as an effective, mainstream method of education and training that provides learning opportunities that are flexible and responsive to learners' needs. Distance learning is now a key component of our new learning society, in which learners must take increased responsibility for control and direction of the learning process (American Council on Education, 2008).

Following Schramm's (1962) conclusions that there was no significant difference in learning between face-to-face and televised learning, researchers compared classroom instruction to other methods of distance education. Numerous studies comparing traditional classroom based instruction with technology-supported instruction have found no significant difference in critical educational variables, such as learning outcomes. Wetzel, Radtke, and Stern (1994) summarized the results of comparative studies until the mid 1990s and also found no significant difference in learning outcomes between the two learning environments. Thomas Russell at North Carolina State University studied hundreds of sources of written material about distance education (Russell, 1998) and concluded that the learning outcomes of students in the traditional classroom are similar to the learning outcomes of students in distance technology classes. Thus, it is called the no significant differences phenomenon.

The American Federation of Teachers and the National Education Association commissioned The Institute of Higher Education Policy to conduct a review of the current research on the effectiveness of distance education to analyze what the research tells us and does not tell us (Merisotis & Phipps, 1999). Merisotis and Phipps (1999) conducted the review of the studies published in the 1990s, and the resultant document is called, "What's the Difference: A Review of Contemporary Research on the Effectiveness of Distance Learning in Education." Overall, students online tended to perform as effectively as traditional students. Online students had similar learning experiences and were as satisfied with their learning experience as traditional students. But the authors noted several shortcomings in the original research: lack of control for extraneous variables; lack of randomization of subjects; questionable validity and reliability of instruments used to measure student outcome and attitude; no control for reactive effects such as the impact of motivation and interest because taking a course online is a novelty. The authors suggest that because of these shortcomings, the conclusions are inconclusive. The question—What is the best way to teach students?—prevails (Merisotis & Phipps, 1999).

Other variables observed with no significant differences between learning environments include overall course satisfaction, course organization, or meeting class objectives. Leasure, Davis, and Thievon (2000) looked at these differences between traditional lecture and distance-based instruction and reported no significant differences. Course satisfaction was evaluated by Allen, Bourhis, and Mabry (2002). These authors conducted a meta-analysis and found no difference in satisfaction levels with a slight preference for traditional face-to-face educational format over a distance-based education format. Researchers began to move beyond comparative studies and into other methods, such as discourse analysis and in-depth interviews. These methods have afforded theoretical frameworks on which to base various studies and have revealed further complexities involved in distance education, such as social, economic, and global issues affecting the field (Saba, 2000).

Chickering and Ehrman (1996) used the American Association for Higher Education's (AAHE) "Principles for Good Practice" to develop best practices to teach students in online environments in a paper called "Implementing the Seven Principles: Technology as Lever." They suggest the following:

1. Good practice encourages contact between students and faculty: asynchronous communication (time delayed) is enhanced by using online environments. Students and faculty exchange work more effectively and safely in online environments than in the traditional classroom. Communication becomes more intimate, protected, and connected online than in face-to-face interaction.

2. Good practice develops reciprocity and cooperation among students: technology provides opportunities for interaction in online learning environments. Students can share their knowledge and experience in small groups, study groups, during group problem solving, and in activities related to learning content. For example, the learning content may be epidemiology and the epidemiologic triangle: the agent, the host, and the environment. Online students can be assigned to small learning groups and given the assignment, "Explain how West Nile virus occurs and develop strategies to prevent it from occurring."

3. Good practice uses active learning techniques: the technology included in online learning systems provides opportunity for active learning. For example, students in an online community health nursing course are given an exercise to assess a community. Students are directed to obtain census and vital

statistics data. Students then view a windshield survey (made by faculty). The exercise is to write a composite picture of the community to share with their learning group. Each small learning group discusses the exercise and develops a composite picture of the commonalties identified by members of the group. The group consensus summary is posted in a public discussion forum for all groups to read.

4. Good practice gives prompt feedback: technology provides many opportunities for feedback, both synchronous (real time, i.e., virtual chat), asynchronous (time delayed, i.e., discussion boards), and e-mail. What is considered "prompt" should be clarified in the course directions or in the syllabus. For example, the instructor might post the following: "I will read all posting on the discussion board once a week and will write a comment to the group." "I will answer all e-mails in three working days." "Office hours: I will be available in the virtual chat room on Wednesday from 7 to 8 p.m. Please join me to ask questions or clarify content."

5. Good practice emphasizes time on task: time is critical and using time wisely is a goal online. Online courses save the student commuting and parking time. Students can learn anywhere—at home or at work, or wherever there is a computer. A rule of thumb is to double or triple the number of course credits to determine the number of hours a week a student will spend online. For example, a student enrolled in a three credit course may spend six to nine hours a week in the online course.

6. Good practice communicates high expectations: some students register for online courses because they think they will be easier. Then they find out that is a fallacy. Expectations should be clear with students. If students are not performing at the expected level, the instructor can e-mail the student and describe observed behavior and delineate expected behavior. For example, the instructor sees that a student is posting such comments as "I agree, Cathy" or "great idea, Michelle." The faculty can send an e-mail saying "Mary, I have read your postings and can see that in

some you clearly express your ideas and you use the literature to support your ideas and in other postings your comments are less substantiated. I can see that you have excellent ideas and would like to see you share these with your peers."

7. Good practice respects diverse talents and ways of learning: the advantage of online courses is the many resources available to accommodate a variety of learning styles. For example, for the visual learners, use PowerPoint. For audio learners, use audio-visual material, and for readers, add notes. Slide shows can be easily constructed for disseminating content online. Links can be added. There can be schedules for students who need structure; for example, each student is expected to post to a discussion at least twice a week.

Billings and Connors (n.d.) applied these best practices to nursing. They suggest a model that focuses on the best practices for technology, faculty, students, and outcomes. They developed a set of examples for each of the areas of focus in the model. For example, a best practice for technology is infrastructure, and the evidence includes access to the Internet, course management software, user support, and appropriate hardware and software.

While the guiding principles of quality practice were being developed, universities were struggling with what Noble (1998) calls automation. According to Noble, automation, "the distribution of digitized course material online, without the participation of professors who develop such material—is often justified as an inevitable part of the new knowledge-based society" (Noble, 1998, p. 1). UCLA instituted the "Instructional Enhancement Initiative," which mandated that all Arts and Sciences courses have a Web-based delivery component. The university partnered with private corporations and formed its own for-profit company (Noble, 1998). Noble says, "It is by no accident that the high-tech transformation of higher education is being initiated and implemented from the top down, either without any student and faculty involvement in the decision-making or despite it" (Noble, 1998, p. 2). Although faculty and students were opposed to the initiative, UCLA administrators continued with their plans (Noble, 1998). Further, Noble (1998) cites a reason for the decision to continue—the fear of being left behind in an academic trend. He calls this "the commercialism of higher education." The function of the university is to teach and universities are developing their courseware into marketable, sellable products in hopes of getting "a piece of the commercial action for their institutions or themselves, as vendors in their own right of software and content" (Noble, 1998, p. 5). The concern of faculty is the quality of education. Faculty view Web-based instruction as commoditizing education, and the fear is that the quality of instruction will be compromised by automation.

Online courses and programs grew from 1999 to 2001 through grants awarded by the Department of Education called "Learning Anytime Anywhere Partnerships" (LAAP) for innovative distance learning partnerships. With funding from President Bill Clinton's Fund for the Improvement of Postsecondary Education, LAAP received $10 million in 1999, $23.3 million in 2000, and $30 million in 2001. The project is being phased out (Carnevale, 2001), but the emphasis on partnerships continued to grow.

CURRENT STATE

The U.S. Census Bureau (2005) has included questions about computer use in their census surveys since 1984 and Internet use since 1997. They found that 62% of U.S. households had computers, and 55% of households had Internet access in 2003. The percentage of children who use the Internet was 42% in 2003 (Child Trends, n.d.). Approximately 91% of children three years of age and older use computers, and 59% use the Internet (Institute of Education Science, 2006). Over 50% of students use home computers to play games; 47% to complete school assignments, and 45% to use the Internet (Institute of Education Science, 2006). According to the Bureau of Labor Statistics in 2003, two of every five employees use the Internet and email at work (Bureau of Labor Statistics, 2005).

How are computers used in teaching and learning? "Campus Computing" is the largest continuing study of the role of computing and information technology in American higher education. Their 2007 survey provided data from 555 public and private colleges and universities throughout the United States (Green, 2007). When asked if computers or PDA handhelds are required or strongly recommended in their schools, 45% of the respondents said yes. When asked if they had preferred provider agreements, 45% had one with Apple and 55% with Dell (Green, 2007). When asked if technology has improved instruction on their campus, 93% agreed or strongly agreed. They report that:

- 39% of the respondent schools use computer-based classrooms labs
- 19% use computer-based simulations/exercises
- 56% use presentation handouts
- 82% use electronic mail
- 32% use commercial courseware/instructional resources
- 60% use Internet resources
- 50% use course management tools for online course resources
- 43% use Web pages for class material and resources
- 5% use a classroom response system (clickers), and
- 2% use podcasting.

"The Horizon Report" (New Media Consortium, 2008) is an annual report that describes emerging technologies that will most likely impact teaching and learning. The top trends for 2008 and the next five years are:

- Use of Web 2.0 and social networking with collective intelligence.
- Work, collaborate, and communicate with more fluid boundaries.
- Use of more powerful and smaller devices that will allow information to be more accessible and portable.
- A widening in the gap between students' and faculty's perceptions of technology.

It is estimated that about 70% of academic leaders believe that student demand for online learning is still growing, and about 83% of institutions who currently offer courses online offerings think that that their enrollments in online courses will increase in the coming year (Online Nation, n.d.).

Technology is changing the way we teach and learn both in the classroom and in online learning environments. How are computers and the Internet used for teaching and learning in nursing? Nurses teach patients who are the consumers of health care, nurses teach their peers through continuing education and nurses teach students.

TEACHING CONSUMERS OF HEALTH CARE

Ferguson (1997, p 251) defines consumer health informatics (CHI) as "the study of consumer interfaces in health care systems" and describes two types: community CHI resources and clinical CHI resources. Community resources are those that consumers can access online. Clinical resources are programs or systems that are provided to selected members or patients, for example, physician-patient e-mail or home health workstations. Ferguson calls health consumers "online self-helpers." Online self-helpers go online looking for information, support, and advice. They get this through online support forums that provide information, asynchronous chat, and live chat (Ferguson, 1997). Ferguson suggests that online self-helpers are able to get answers to their own questions, answers to other self-helpers' questions, and general information.

Ferguson (1997) concluded that one of the roots of our current health care crisis is our current "professional-as-authority" model of health care. Ferguson (1997) cites two laws that will predict the future. The first is Moore's Law—computers will expand exponentially with a resultant increase in bandwidth and decrease in cost. The second is Metcalf's Law—the number of computer networks will increase exponentially as the number of people who connect to the network increases. Because of the current trend toward acceptance of online health information, Ferguson (1997) predicts a major transformation will take place that will redefine health care. This prediction is supported by Eysenbach and Diepgen (2001), who describe the convergence of several factors that came together at the same time to promote and expand e-health. Consumers became more responsible for their own health care at a time when health providers realized the potential of having their consumers gain information and support online. The value of an educated, empowered consumer in improving the quality of health care is recognized. During a time when the cost of health care is an issue, online learning has cost-saving benefits in that consumers can access information and support online. The information age and consumerism have merged to empower consumers through access to quality health care information on the web.

Leaffer and Gonda (2000) titled their journal article, "The Internet: An Underutilized Tool in Patient Education." The title summarized their study findings that when senior citizens were taught how to use the Internet to search, find, and share health information, 66% continued this behavior in a 90-day follow-up, and 47% continued to search for health information after the study ended. The senior citizens who used the Internet to find health information reported more satisfaction with health care as a result of the increased knowledge and discussion with their physician. These findings are relevant to nursing.

Nursing has traditionally played a strong role in patient education, which now incorporates Internet technology. Nursing curricula needs to be reengineered to incorporate the Internet as a valuable patient education tool in order to prepare both nursing students and nurse practitioners for the health care demands of the twenty-first century. The reengineered curricula will have to consider the significant increase in the number of older patients the nursing profession will serve (Leaffer & Gonda, 2000). Nurses should refer seniors to the Internet to search and find credible health information. Nursing faculty should use the Internet to access health information for nursing curricula, and student nurses should be taught how to use the Internet as a source of health information and to teach clients to use the Internet effectively to obtain information. The retrieved information should be critically evaluated by the nurse to ensure its credibility.

Teaching Peers through Continuing Education and Training

Telecommunications and distance technologies are transforming how we deliver education and training, because they allow for expanding capacity to respond to the requirements for keeping health professionals up to date. With a long history of serving isolated and remote learners, distance learning has now emerged as an effective, mainstream method of education and training that provides flexible learning opportunities in response to learners' needs. In the past twenty years, physicians, nurses and other health care professionals have continued to seek available technology-supported Continuing Medical Education (CME) for its convenience and accessibility. In a 1998 article Plank writes, "if the Internet is not recognized and used for educational purposes by nurses, those nurses will be left behind" (p. 166). The Internet offers "a unique opportunity to provide innovative approaches to career mobility for registered nurses" (O'Brien & Renner, 2000, p.13), because the Internet provides a cost-effective and accessible method of imparting information to nurses. The challenges are that the nurses need to have (or learn) technical skills and communication skills to interact online.

A recent comprehensive review of CME available on the Web found that the number of sites offering Web-based CME had risen 18% between 2003 and 2006 (Sklar, 2006). CME Web (the largest source for online CME), accredited by the ACCME, offers 885 courses and over 800 hours of continuing education credit annually.

What do medical professionals think is important in CME courses? In a review of 30 CME courses, quality of content was the characteristic most important to participants, and too little interaction was the largest source of dissatisfaction (Casebeer, Kristofco, Strasser, 2004). Cobb (2004) summarized the findings of nine distance CME studies and found that the majority of respondents thought that the distance format was effective in imparting new knowledge. The advantages (Bergren, 1999) cited by school nurses are that they can learn at their own pace and on their own schedule, and they can learn about topics of importance and interest to them. The Internet is an option for certification review courses. Family or Adult Nurse Practitioner Certification Examination review courses online offer the nurse guidance and support through interactive learning, audiovisual presentations, exercises, practice tests, and links to resources.

Research suggests that distance CME can be effective but it is the design of these courses that needs to be carefully scrutinized for optimal learning opportunities and optimal delivery of content.

TEACHING NURSING STUDENTS

The American Association of Colleges of Nursing (AACN) approved a white paper, "Distance Technology in Nursing Education," developed by the AACN Task Force on Distance Technology and Nursing Education on July 26, 1999. The importance of technology in nursing education was recognized. The focus of the white paper was using technology to enhance nursing education. To do so, schools must strategically plan for distance education programs. Several factors need to be addressed by nursing educators and other leaders in education and health care institutions, as well as by external funders and policy makers:

- Superior distance education programs require substantial institutional financial investment in equipment, infrastructure, and faculty development.
- Local, regional, and national planning for multisite communications needs to consider coordination of services, compatibility, and progressive upgrading of hardware, as well as policies that lower transmission costs within and across state lines.
- The use of distance technology and, in particular, Web-based media, has raised questions regarding intellectual property and copyrights, privacy of educational dialogue, and other related legal and ethical issues that require continued clarification.
- Technology-mediated teaching strategies can dramatically change the way teaching and learning occurs, challenging the traditional relationship of students to academic institutions. These strategies may change conventional thinking about how quality of educational programs is assessed and what is required to support student learning (e.g., library access, counseling services, computing equipment, tuition, and financial aid).

Distance education technology has provided some nursing schools an advantage in recruiting students and is increasing competition among institutions (American Association of Colleges of Nursing, 1999).

The AACN (2000a) outlines differences in distance education from traditional learning in nursing. In distance education, student and faculty roles change. The teacher moves from sage-on-the-stage to guide-on-the-side, and students interact more and become more cohesive. Distance learning is a strategy that will boost enrollment in schools of nursing (American Association of Colleges of Nursing 2000a; 2000b), because it will attract students who would not enroll in traditional programs, with the result that many Registered Nurse (RN) to Bachelor of Science in Nursing (BSN) curricula are offered online. Distance education gives faculty an opportunity to use technology to teach in new and creative ways. Distance education can open the doors to more collaboration through partnerships to share resources and faculty expertise.

In summary, technology is an integral part of teaching. Technology has evolved from print to television to online. Computers and the Internet are at home, at work, and in schools. Teaching with technology has best practices for both education and for nursing. The best practices are the basis for developing quality learning environments for students, consumers, and medical professionals.

Whether the nurse is developing an intranet site, orienting new nurses, updating skills for nurses, teaching consumers, teaching student nurses, or developing continuing education programs in online environments, a basic set of skills are necessary. Those skills include:

- Having an understanding of the impact of infrastructure, resources, and support systems in imparting information and communicating online.
- Understanding pedagogy in order to make decisions about what to teach and how to teach it effectively.
- Having knowledge and skills in technology to be able to develop Web sites and put information online.
- Reconceptualizing learning to online environments.
- Using pedagogy and technology to design creative, effective learning environments online.

- Teaching and communicating in online environments.
- Assessing and evaluating learning online.

With basic knowledge and understanding of these skills, the nurse can begin to effectively create quality online learning environment.

REFERENCES

Allen, M., Bourhis, J., Burrell, N., & Mabry, E. (2002). Comparing student satisfaction with distance education to traditional classrooms in higher education: A meta-analysis. *American Journal of Distance Education*, 16(2), 83–97.

American Association of Colleges of Nursing. (1999, July). *AACN white paper: Distance technology in nursing education.* Retrieved April 16, 2008, from http://www.aacn. nche.edu/Publications/WhitePapers/whitepaper.htm

American Association of Colleges of Nursing. (2000a). *Distance learning is changing and challenging nursing education.* Retrieved April 16, 2008, from http://www.aacn. nche.edu/publications/issues/jan2000.htm

American Association of Colleges of Nursing. (2000b). Amid nursing shortages, schools employ strategies to boost enrollment. Retrieved April 16, 2008, from http://www. aacn.nche.edu/Publications/issues/ib600wb.htm

American Council on Education. (2008). Center for adult learning. Retrieved April 16, 2008, from http://www.acenet.edu/Content/NavigationMenu/ProgramsServices/ Adults/adults11.htm

Bergren, M. D. (1999). Online continuing education. *Journal of School Nursing,* 15(4), 32–34.

Billings, B. & Connors, H. (n.d.). Best practices in online learning. Retrieved on April 21, 2008, from http://www.electronicvision.com/nln/chapter02/index.htm

Bureau of Labor Statistics. (2005). Computer and Internet use at work. Retrieved February 15, 2008, from http://www.bls.gov/home.htm

Carnevale, D. (2001). Education Department cuts new distance-education grants. *Chronicle of Higher Education,* September 28.

Casebeer, L., Kristofco, R., Strasser, S. (2004). Standardizing evaluation of on-line continuing medical education: Physician knowledge, attitudes, and reflection on practice. *Journal of Continuing Education in the Health Professions,* 24, 68–75.

Chickering, A. W. & Ehrmann, S. C. (1996). *AAHE Bulletin, October.* Retrieved April 3, 2008, from http://www.tltgroup.org/programs/seven.html

Child Trends. (n.d.). Data Bank. Retrieved on March 1, 2008 from http://www. childtrendsdatabank.org/indicators/69homecomputeruse.cfm

Cobb, S. (2004). Internet continuing education for health care professionals: An integrative review. *Journal of Continuing Education in the Health Professions,* 24, 171–180.

Eysenbach, G. & Diepgen, T. (2001). The role of e-health and consumer health informatics for evidence-based patient choice in the 21st century. *Clinics in Dermatology,* 19, 11–17.

Ferguson, T. (1997). Health online and the empowered medical consumer. *Journal on Quality Improvement,* 23(5), 251–257.

Green, K. (2007). Campus Computing 2007. Encino, CA: The Campus Computing Project.

Institute of Education Science. (2006). Computer and Internet use by students in 2003. Retrieved on March 1, 2008, from http://nces.ed.gov/Pubsearch/pubsinfo. asp?pubid=2006065

Instructional Technology Council (n.d.). Retrieved on February 5, 2008, from http://144.162.197.250/definition.htm

Leaffer, T. & Gonda, B. (2000). The Internet: An underutilized tool in patient education. *Computers in Nursing,* 18(1), 47–52.

Leasure, A., Davis, L., & Thievon, S. (2000). Comparison of student outcomes and preferences in a traditional vs. World Wide Web-based baccalaureate nursing research course. *Journal of Nursing Education,* 39(4), 149–54.

Martyn, M. (2007). Clickers in the classroom: an active learning approach. Retrieved on March 15, 2008, from http://www.educause.edu/ir/library/pdf/eqm0729.pdf

Merisotis, J. P. & Phipps, R. A. (1999). What's the difference? A review of contemporary research on the effectiveness of distance learning in higher education. Washington D.C.: The Institute for Higher Education Policy.

New Media Consortium. (2008). The Horizon Report: 2008 Edition. Retrieved April 2, 2008, from http://www.educause.edu/ir/library/pdf/CSD5320.pdf

Noble, D. F. (1998). Digital diploma mills: The automation of higher education. *The MIT Press,* 86, 107–117.

O'Brien, B. S. & Renner, A. (2000). Nurses online: Career mobility for registered nurses. *Journal of Professional Nursing,* 16(1), 13–20.

Plank, K. P. (1998). Nursing on-line for continuing education credit. *Journal of Continuing Education in Nursing,* 29(4), 165–172.

Russell, T. (1998). *No significant difference: Phenomenon as reported in 248 research reports, summaries, and papers* (4th ed.). Raleigh: North Carolina State University.

Saba, F. (2000). Research in distance education: A status report. *International Review of Research in Open and Distance Learning.* Retrieved April 21, 2008, from http://www.irrodl.org/index.php/irrodl/article/viewArticle/4

Schramm, W. (1962). What we know about learning from instructional television. In *Educational television: The next ten years.* Stanford, CA: The Institute for Communication Research, Stanford University.

Simulation Labs. (2004). Retrieved on March 15, 2008 from http://nursing.umaryland. edu/docs/csl/Pulse-article-2004.pdf

Sklar, B. (2006). Online CME: An update. Retrieved April 22, 2008, from http://www.cmelist.com/mastersthesis

Wetzel, D., Radtke, P., & Stern, H. (1994). Instructional effectiveness of video media. Hillsdale, NJ: Lawrence Earlbaum Associates.

U.S. Census Bureau. (2005). Computer and Internet Use in the United States: 2003. Retrieved April 21, 2008, from http://www.census.gov/prod/2005pubs/p23-208.pdf

Williams, M. L., Paprock, K. & Covington B. (1999). Distance learning. The essential guide. London: Sage Publications.

Woods, R., & Baker, J. (2004). Interaction and immediacy in online learning. *International review of research in open and distance learning,* 5(2), 1–13.

2

Pedagogy Associated with Learning in Online Environments

CAROL A. O'NEIL

Technology can reach a broad range of students and thus has expanded access to education. Making nursing education more accessible is important for two reasons: alleviating the nursing shortage and increasing the number of BSN-prepared nurses. Potential nursing students may be employed full time and may have families. As a result, they may not have time to attend traditional education programs. By providing online learning environments and thereby enhancing access, more students may enroll in nursing education programs, thus reducing the nursing shortage. To meet the complex demands of today's health care environment, a federal advisory panel has recommended that by 2010 at least two thirds of the basic nurse workforce hold baccalaureate or higher degrees in nursing. Aware of this need, RNs are seeking the BSN degree in increasing numbers (American Association of Colleges of Nursing, 2001).

Graduate students also can take courses and programs over the Internet through online universities such as Walden (www.waldenu. edu/c/Schools/Schools_9188.htm) and Excelsior (www.excelsior.edu/ Excelsior_College/School_Of_Nursing) and through public and private colleges and universities who offer programs, both degree and certificate, online. For example, the University of Maryland School of Nursing (nursing.umaryland.edu) offers their Graduate Informatics and Health Services and Leadership and Management master's program and their Teaching and Learning in Nursing and Health Professions certificate program online. The University of Arizona School of Nursing (www.nursing.arizona.edu/Doctoral.htm) offers their PhD program online. To meet increased demand for online learning opportunities, partnerships among universities and health care institutions have developed to allow for the sharing of resources and to enhance the quality of online learning in both national and international perspectives.

ONLINE AND FACE-TO-FACE LEARNING ENVIRONMENTS

What are the differences between online and face-to-face learning environments? The online learning environment is accessible anytime and anywhere, which makes it convenient for the learner. Online learning is dependent only on technology: if the technology is available, so is the education. Face-to-face learning is scheduled, and classes are offered at set times in specific places. The course a learner needs may only be offered 50 miles away at 8 a.m. The student must be available when and where the course is offered. Face-to-face learning tends to be a one-size-fits-all approach, with lecture as the major teaching modality.

In an online learning environment, students can log on and review their course material whenever they want and wherever a computer with Internet access is available. Online students are spared driving to class during winter months in snowy locations. They are also spared the inconvenience of traffic, the scarcity and cost of parking, and the worry of compromised safety, especially when taking night classes in cities.

Since learning online is technology dependent, the GIGO rule applies: Garbage In—Garbage Out. Online learning is not "slapping classroom content online." The positive resources of technology are used to bring content and experiences to learners. In other words, the resource is used to enrich the content. Learning online can be seen as a lonely and isolated experience, because online learners cannot see each other, and the teacher cannot see the students. "If you can't see them, you can't teach them," seems to be a traditionalist mantra. Going back to GIGO, online education that excludes interaction denies the learner a quality learning experience. Online learners should be actively interacting with each other (student to student) and with teachers (student to teacher).

Cincinnati State Technical and Community College (2004) offers these as advantages of an online course:

- Online learning offers a tremendous opportunity to learn without the limitations of time or location. Students have the flexibility to learn any time, anywhere.
- Contrary to popular opinion, distance learning can be more personal and interactive than traditional classroom courses. Students who are uncomfortable asking questions in class can communicate more comfortably with faculty.
- Students often have the opportunity to learn according to their preferred learning styles.
- Students become more self-directed and responsible for their own learning. (Cincinnati State Technical and Community College, 2004).

CHARACTERISTICS OF ONLINE COURSES

The online learning experience consists of an audience, a purpose, learning objectives, content, multimedia design, interaction (synchronous and asynchronous), and assessment and evaluation activities. In an online learning module, there are objectives that tell the learner what he or she will accomplish and guide the design of the course. In addition, orientation and support services are provided for teachers and learners. A learning module should be about 50% self-study and 50% interaction. The format for the learner is read the material, do the assignments (activities), discuss the assignments, and then report on the assignment.

The Illinois Online Network (2007) outlines an online program's key elements: the students, the curriculum, the facilitator, and the technology. A student must have a positive attitude, technology skills, and commitment to be a good candidate for online learning. Courses should be organized and should focus on applying what is learned to the real world. The material should foster critical thinking and the exchange of ideas with students and faculty. An online curriculum should integrate life, work, and educational experience; include ample time for the completion of the assigned work; utilize a minimal amount of memorization; maintain a balance between the technology, the facilitator and the students; and incorporate group and team activities. The learning outcomes must be achievable and offer the opportunity for students to use them in practical, everyday situations (ION, 2007).

The facilitator is responsible for the appropriate design of the curriculum and for facilitation of the course. Technology is a tool for learning and it should be user-friendly, reliable, accessible, and affordable. The technology should accommodate the lowest common denominator of the class.

According to the University of Maryland University College (n.d.), typical elements of learning online include an asynchronous quality, frequent participation with faculty and students, lectures and assigned readings, individual and group classes, use of library resources, and proctored quizzes and exams.

The National Education Association (n.d.) lists the following Core Beliefs on Effective Education Online:

- Are instructor-led, student-centered, collaborative, and flexible
- Foster information, communication, and technology
- Have clear and concise expectations and instructions
- Account for learning style
- Use best practices

Pedagogy

Pedagogy is the theory, methods, and activities for maximizing teaching and learning. Bill Pelz (2004) identified the following three principles of effective online pedagogy:

Principle #1: Let the students do (most of) the work.

Principle #2: Interactivity is the heart and soul of effective asynchronous learning.

Principle #3: Strive for presence.

His belief is that the pedagogy of learning online is grounded in student-centered learning and in employing active learning activities. Interactivity is essential for learning online and the presence of both faculty and students is essential for effective online learning.

Pedagogy includes consideration of the influences of developmental level and learning style on learning and the learning theories upon which online learning environments are created.

Influences on Learning: Developmental Level—Adult Learning

Online learners are adults, and an effective instructor needs to understand how adults learn. Compared to children and teens, adults have special needs and requirements as learners. Adult learning is not a unique and specific process. Instead it is a set of generalizations about "the adult learner" that imply that people within a certain, yet-to-be-defined age range form a homogenous group. But differences of culture, cognitive style, life experiences, and gender may be far more important to learning than age (Shannon, 2003).

Malcolm Knowles (1970) pioneered the field of adult learning and identified adult learning characteristics that should be appropriately incorporated into the development of education. Knowles found that adults are autonomous and self-directed. Their teachers must actively involve adult participants in the learning process and serve as facilitators for them. Specifically, they must get the participants' perspectives about what topics to cover and let them work on projects that reflect their interests. They should allow the participants to assume responsibility for presentations and group leadership. They have to be sure to act as facilitators, guiding participants to their own knowledge rather than supplying them with facts. Finally, they must show participants how the class will help them reach their goals. Adults have accumulated a wealth of life experiences and knowledge that may include work-related activities, family responsibilities, and previous education. Adult learners need to connect learning to this knowledge and experience base. To help them do so, teachers should draw out participants' experience and knowledge that is relevant to the topic. Educators relate theories and concepts to the participants and recognize the value of experience in learning.

Knowles identified another characteristic of adults: they are goal-oriented. Upon enrolling in a course, adult learners usually know what goal they want to attain. Therefore they appreciate an educational program that is organized and has clearly defined elements. Instructors must show participants how this class will help them attain their goals and must ensure that the course is relevant and practical. Learning should be applicable to their work or other responsibilities to be of value to them. In adulthood, learning is best achieved when the subject matter is presented in an authentic learning environment.

Instructors must relate the relevance of the lesson to the learner's job. Instructors must show adult learners respect and acknowledge the wealth of experiences these students bring to the classroom. These adults should be treated as equals in experience and knowledge and allowed to voice their opinions freely in class. Because of these characteristics, adult-learning programs should capitalize on the experience of the participants, and they should adapt to the aging range of the participants. Additionally, the course offerings should consider advanced stages of participant development by offering as much choice as possible in the organization of the learning program.

Influences on Learning: Learning Style

Learning styles are simply different ways in which we think and learn. Understanding and addressing learning styles when preparing instructional materials will enhance the entire teaching and learning process. There are many approaches to identifying learning styles. The four most widely recognized methods of assessing learning style are: VARK, Index of Learning Style, Multiple Intelligences, and Myers-Briggs Type Indicator.

The VARK (www.vark-learn.com/english/index.asp) is a 13-item online questionnaire that provides users with a profile of their visual, auditory, or kinesthetic preferences. "Let me see it!" exemplifies the visual learner; "Just tell me!" exemplifies the auditory learner, and "Let me do it!" is the kinesthetic learner.

The Index of Learning Style (www.engr.ncsu.edu/learning-styles/ilsweb.html) is a 44-item online questionnaire that assesses preferences on these four dimensions: active/reflective, sensing/intuitive, visual/verbal, and sequential/global. Active learners prefer to apply learning, and reflective learners prefer to think about learning. Sensing learners like to learn facts, while intuitive learners like to learn through discovery. The visual learner learns by seeing, while the verbal learner learns by hearing. Sequential learners are linear and logical and learn in steps, and global learners learn by seeing the big picture first and then by seeing the component parts.

Howard Gardner, developer of the Multiple Intelligences theory, describes nine intelligences. Thirteen Ed Online (Educational Broadcasting Company, 2004) provides an online workshop for "Tapping into Multiple Intelligences" and a comprehensive "Multiple Intelligence Inventory" (with 80 questions). The intelligences and definitions of Gardner's Multiple Intelligences are:

- Verbal-Linguistic Intelligence: well-developed verbal skills and sensitivity to the sounds, meanings, and rhythms of words
- Mathematical-Logical Intelligence: ability to think conceptually and abstractly and capacity to discern logical or numerical patterns
- Musical Intelligence: ability to produce and appreciate rhythm, pitch, and timber
- Visual-Spatial Intelligence: capacity to think in images and pictures, to visualize accurately and abstractly
- Bodily-Kinesthetic Intelligence: ability to control one's body movements and to handle objects skillfully
- Interpersonal Intelligence: capacity to detect and respond appropriately to the moods, motivations, and desires of others.

- Intrapersonal Intelligence: capacity to be self-aware and in tune with inner feelings, values, beliefs, and thinking processes
- Naturalist Intelligence: ability to recognize and categorize plants, animals, and other objects in nature
- Existential Intelligence: sensitivity and capacity to tackle deep questions about human existence, such as the meaning of life, why do we die, and how did we get here (Educational Broadcasting Company, 2004)

Meacham (2003) suggests characteristics and learning strategies for each of the learning styles, as outlined in Table 2.1.

The Myers-Briggs Type Indicator (MBTI) is a method of assessing learning style as inferred from a personality inventory. It provides data on four sets of preferences. These preferences result in 16 learning styles, or types. A type is the combination of the four preferences. Myers-Briggs Type Indicator is a widely used and useful instrument when trying to understand of the role of individual differences in the learning process. MBTI (www.humanmetrics.com/cgi-win/JTypes2.asp) scores indicate one's preference on each of following four dimensions:

Extroversion (E) prefers direct attention toward the external world of people and thing

Introversion (I) prefers direct attention toward the inner world of concepts and ideas

Sensing (S) prefers perceiving the world through directly observing the surrounding tangible reality

Intuition (N) prefers perceiving the world through impressions and imagining possibilities

The "Teaching Notes" article from the Georgia State University's Master Teacher Program (n.d.) discusses the four dichotomies underlying the Myers-Briggs Type Indicator (MBTI) and several teaching approaches that will appeal to different MBTI profiles.

Table 2.1

EXAMPLES OF LEARNING STRATEGIES BASED ON MULTIPLE INTELLIGENCES

MULTIPLE INTELLIGENCE	CHARACTERISTICS	LEARNING STRATEGIES
Visual/spatial intelligence	These learners tend to think in pictures	Charts, maps, visuals, metaphors, graphs, diagrams.
Verbal/linguistic intelligence	They learn by speaking and listening	Stories, notes, reading, memorizing, analyzing case studies, text.
Logical/mathematical intelligence	They use reason and logic, and ask "why?"	Spreadsheets, experiments, interviewing, classifying and organizing, developing theories, solving problems.
Bodily/kinesthetic intelligence	These learners have the ability to control body movements and handle physical objects. They interact with the space around them.	Hands-on manipulation, watching videos or presentations, simulations, games, videoconferencing, creating something with hands.
Musical/rhythmical intelligence	Appreciates and products music in sounds, rhythms, and patterns.	Compose songs, tones, and sound effects.
Interpersonal intelligence	These learners have an advanced ability to relate to and understand the feelings of others.	Telling stories about how other people feel, learning teams, small group discussion, role-playing, analyzing case studies, consensus or agreement building exercises.
Intrapersonal intelligence	These learners exhibit a strong sense of self and the ability to understand and share their inner thoughts and feelings.	Surveys, role playing, discussion.
Naturalist intelligence	These learners have an appreciation for and an understanding of the world around them.	Like the outdoors and animals, explore, investigate, field trips, tours

THEORIES IN EDUCATION

Distance based learning is a complex event that cannot be explained with a single learning theory according to Johnson and Aragon (2003). Instead, quality learning environments should be based on instructional principles that are derived from multiple learning theories.

Theories about learning are mostly derived from psychology. While psychology describes how people act, educational theory describes how people learn. We can therefore use educational theories to design and implement effective educational programs.

Behavioral Theory

Behaviorism was one of the most influential theories in the fields of education and psychology. Ivan Pavlov (1849–1936) conducted experiments in Russia with dogs. He rang a bell and then gave the dogs food. He repeated the ringing of the bell and the giving of food over and over until the dogs began to salivate in anticipation of food when the bell rang. This stimulus-response behavior is called classical conditioning. Edward Thorndike (1874–1949) applied behaviorism to education at Columbia University in New York. He postulated that learning was the resultant connection between a stimulus and a response. John B. Watson, who is often referred to as the true father of behaviorism, earned his PhD at the University of Chicago in 1903. Watson's research connected conditioned fear and emotional response.

B.F. Skinner (1904–1990) continued work with stimulus-response but focused on studying voluntary responses. He rewarded responses that were desirable and punished or ignored undesirable responses. His work is called operant conditioning. His theory, like those of Pavlov, Thorndike, and Watson, was based on behavioral change while mental processes were ignored. Behavioral change is what is observed—for example, what one says or does, or how one behaves. If a behavior is observed, it is the response to a stimulus. A stimulus is defined as an object in the environment that poses a physiologic threat. A response is anything that one does in response to a stimulus. It could be as simple as a turn of the head, a twitch, or saying,

"I am sorry," or as complex as designing a building or writing a book. Behaviorism was popular until the 1950s, but it began to lose supporters because the theory explained learning from only a behavioral perspective and is therefore limited in scope.

The psychological theory of behaviorism is used as an educational theory when the learning experience is based on a stimulus and a response and by rewarding behavior that will meet the educational goal and ignoring (or correcting) behavior that is not goal directed.

In behavioral theory, large tasks are broken down into smaller tasks, and each task is learned in successive order. The process is called successive approximations. Traditional learning labs are an example of behaviorist theory, and one nursing example is learning the correct procedure for a dry, sterile dressing. By taking the entire procedure and breaking it down into steps, learners master the first step then move to successive steps until they master every step to complete the procedure. The first step would be to verify the order, then gather equipment, and then prepare the client, set up the area for a sterile field, etc. By learning a segment at a time and doing each segment correctly, the student will be able to successfully complete the dry sterile dressing procedure by putting the learned steps together.

Constructivist Theory

Some educators believe that the teacher can impart information, but that does not mean that the student will learn. These educators believe that learning occurs when the learner uses information to think. Thinking inspires learning. Thinking is stimulated through activities. It is the teacher who provides the content and the activities that initiate and motivate the learners to involve themselves in the activities and thus to think. Thinking helps learners transform information to their context or to a context personal to them and thus see ways to use the information in their lives. Learning becomes the responsibility of the learner.

Jonassen, Peck, Wilson, and Pfeiffer (1998) contrast traditional learning and constructivism. In traditional learning, knowledge is transmitted and is external to the learner, whereas in constructivist learning knowledge is constructed by the learner's action, experience, and perceptions. In traditional learning methods, learning is the transfer of knowledge from the teacher to the student with an emphasis on the outcome. Constructivist learning focuses on interpreting the world and constructing meaning. Learning is active and reflective, which means that there is doing, then reflecting about the doing, and then rethinking about the doing. Action and reflection enable the student to integrate new knowledge with existing knowledge and experiences so that complex mental models can form. Integrating the old and the new learning allows the student to look at the world from a unique perspective. Learning is authentic and resembles real-life experiences.

Constructivist learning is process oriented with an emphasis on collaboration and conversation among learners and teachers. Instruction also differs. In the traditional classroom, instruction is the imparting of information from the top down using a deductive thinking process. Learning is competitive and is controlled by the instructor. In the constructivist approach instruction is inductive, from the bottom up. Learning opportunities are diverse and increase in complexity. The instructor is a model and a coach who encourages exploration of ideas, and learning is learner-centered and learner-generated.

Constructivism assumes that learning is personal and that the student brings past knowledge and experience to the learning situation. Constructivism is the process of bringing new knowledge to past experiences to construct a new reality and to make sense and meaning out of the world. How do students construct their own reality? It is through engaging in an active learning process. Active learning is an approach that engages the student in thinking and rethinking, thus creating new ideas. Students interact with the environment (content, faculty, activities, peers). Active learning, according to Dodge (n.d.), involves the process of providing students with situations that require them to read, speak, listen, think, and write. Although lectures may be well-written and well-delivered, they often pass from the ear to the hand, leaving the mind untouched. The active learning process places responsibility on the learners themselves and lends itself to a wider range of learning styles.

Active learning on the Web involves taking a critical look at the resources that already exist and incorporating them into the learning environment. Examples might include Web quests or newsgroups that would require learners to research information, then return to the online class environment to further collaborate and expand on their research findings. If the student constructs meaning from content, faculty, activities, and peers, then learning environments must be rich with strategies and resources. Technology can provide the richness constructivist learning environments need to guide knowledge construction. Construction of knowledge is the result of social interaction.

Social Interaction

Social interaction has long been thought to increase collaboration and therefore result in increased learning. Jung, Choi, Lim, and Leem (2002) studied interactions in groups and learning outcomes and concluded that adult learners who engaged in social interaction with their instructors and collaborative interaction with peers scored higher on outcome measures of learning than adult learners who did not engage in social and collaborative interaction. This interaction has been recognized as one of the most important components of learning experiences both in conventional education and distance education (Vygotsky, 1978; Moore, 1993).

Research findings suggest that learning in groups improves students' achievement of learning objectives. Vygotsky believed that cognitive development and learning are dependent on social interaction. The major theme of this theoretical framework is that social interaction plays a fundamental role in the process of learning. A second aspect of Vygotsky's theory is the idea that the potential for cognitive development is limited to a certain "time span" which he refers to as the zone of proximal development (ZPD). It is during this time that consciousness is raised and a range of skills can be developed with adult guidance or peer collaboration. Vygotsky's methods of analysis and conclusions about the development of human thought and language are still accurate today and can be applied to the study of computer mediated communication (Bacalarski, n.d.).

Little investigation, however, has been done to compare the effects of different types of interaction (peer to peer, student to instructor) on learning in distance learning environments.

One study (Fulford and Zhang, 1993) did look at learner perception of interaction in learning and concluded that perception of the level of interaction is a critical predictor of learner satisfaction. These authors stated that overall interaction dynamics may have a stronger impact on learners' satisfaction than strictly personal participation. Interestingly, it was also found that vicarious interaction may also result in greater learner satisfaction than the divided attention necessary to ensure the overt engagement of each participant. The ramification of this finding is that online instructors should devise strategies to increase and improve learners' perception of overall interaction.

TECHNOLOGY AND LEARNING

Technology has traditionally been used for the purpose of conveying information to students. Jonassen, Peck, Wilson, and Pfeiffer (1998) suggest that technology does more—that technology can be used to support the student's creation of meaning out of learning. Technology can foster learning because:

- Technology is a tool that can be used to support knowledge construction. Technology allows students to share knowledge and experience and build mental models.
- Technology is an information vehicle for exploring knowledge to support learning-by-constructing. Technology allows access to information and databases from which to acquire knowledge.
- Technology supports learning by doing. Technology supports real-world simulations and case studies. Technology provides an opportunity for students to learn from and resolve these scenarios in a safe, supportive environment.
- Technology is a social medium that supports student learning by conversing. Through synchronous and asynchronous learning, students can discuss and build consensus.

■ Technology is an intellectual partner that supports learning by reflecting. Technology can provide learners with ways to articulate and represent what they know.

So, how can we bring developmental theory, learning style, learning theory, and technology together to create effective learning environments? Undergraduate nursing education traditionally includes faculty-developed behavioral objectives, with content developed by faculty to meet the objectives and evaluation that focuses on the attainment of objectives. This faculty-centered approach is an example of behaviorism. The teacher is responsible for focusing on:

■ Identification of relevant stimuli and response
■ Identification of the learner's entry level and the setting of student expectations
■ Analysis of learner skills and knowledge, developmental level, and learning style
■ Planning a reinforcement schedule
■ Constant confirmation of expectations; maintenance of motivation
■ Development of individualized instruction and exercises
■ Constant assessment of learning each skill before progressing to another skill.

The student's role is to achieve the objectives. Nursing uses objectives to guide and evaluate learning, and objectives are an integral component of nursing education and training. Here is the dilemma: behaviorism is teacher-centered, and online learning should be student-centered. Nursing education and training tends toward behaviorism, and the literature supports constructivism as the online approach to effective learning. If teacher-centered objectives and evaluation of outcomes are necessities, techniques can be used to make the behaviorist favor constructivist components and thereby become more student-centered. One technique is to include assessments of student learning styles and structured learning experiences to accommodate those learning styles. Once a student's learning style is assessed, develop a prescriptive plan for each student to guide their learning. Objectives can be written in a behavioral format, but students can provide real-life case studies to analyze and thus meet objectives. When a combination of behaviorist and constructivist approaches are used, the learning is called a "guided constructivist learning model."

If guided constructivism were the theory used to design online learning environments, objectives would be teacher centered and would guide the learning experience. Emphasis would be placed on the process of knowledge construction rather than on the outcomes of learning. Content would be presented to accommodate various learning styles and developmental levels, and an emphasis would be placed on active learning through questions, case studies, and projects that would help the student develop mental models and test reality. These approaches would allow the student to apply basic information to real world practice.

SUCCESSFUL ONLINE STUDENTS

Successful online students have common characteristics:

- They are highly motivated, independent, and active learners.
- They have good organizational and time management skills.
- They are disciplined to study without external reminders.
- They are able to adapt to new learning environments.

The Illinois Online Network (2007) suggests that the students who most benefit from online learning live long distances from the campus and have busy lives with families, a profession, and other responsibilities. The successful student is mature, open-minded, self-motivated, accepting of critical thinking, willing to work collaboratively, has good written communication skills, and has a minimum level of technological experience.

What are the providers of online learning telling their potential students about what makes a successful online student? Included in the online resource material for Illinois Online Network (2007), is a list of qualities that includes:

- Be open-minded about sharing life, work, and educational experiences as part of the learning process.
- Be able to communicate through writing and be willing to "speak up" if problems arise.
- Be self-motivated, self-disciplined, and willing and able to commit to 4 to 15 hours per week per course. Accept critical thinking and decision making as part of the learning process.
- Have access to a computer and a modem.
- Be able to think ideas through before responding.
- Feel that high quality learning can take place without going to a traditional classroom.

How to Prepare to Be a Successful Online Student (eLearners.com, LLC, 1999–2007) is a resource guide for such topics as: setting up a home office, writing A+ discussion question answers, avoiding the feeling of isolation, and other topics.

In summary, learning in online environments is an educational methodology that is most effective when the developmental level and learning styles of a student are assessed and a theory is chosen to organize learning. Online learning is best organized by using constructivist learning theory. Nursing traditionally uses behavioral objectives to guide learning. Online learning in nursing can use a constructivist approach but must also include behaviorism; thus the term guided constructivism is used to describe teaching and learning nursing online. The successful online student organizes learning time and space, schedules time to study, and interacts with other students and faculty formally and informally.

REFERENCES

American Association of Colleges of Nursing (2001). Strategies to reverse the new nursing shortage. Retrieved on February 27, 2008, from http://www.aacn.nche.edu/Publications/positions/tricshortage.htm

Bacalarski, M. (n.d.). Vygotski's developmental theories and the adulthood of computer-mediated communication: A comparison and an illumination. Retrieved on February 26, 2008, from http://psych.hanover.edu/vygotsky/bacalar.html

Cincinnati State Technical and Community College (2004). Advantages of online learning. Retrieved on February 23, 2008 from http://www.cincinnatistate.edu/CurrentStudent/Academics/AcademicDivisions/About_DL.htm

Dodge, B. (no date). Active learning on the web. Retrieved February 27, 2008 from http://edweb.sdsu.edu/people/bdodge/Active/ActiveLearning.html

Educational Broadcasting Company. (2004). Concept to classroom: Tapping into Multiple Intelligences. Retrieved on April 15, 2008, from http://www.thirteen.org/edonline/concept2class/mi/index.html

eLearners.com, LLC (1999–2007). How to be a successful online student. Retrieved February 27, 2008 from http://www.elearners.com/guide/how-to-be-a-successful-online-student.pdf

Fulford, C. P., & Zhang, S. (1993). Perceptions of interaction: The critical predictor in distance education. *American Journal of Distance Education, 7*(3), 8–21.

Georgia State University Master Teacher Program (n.d.). Teaching students with different learning styles. Retrieved June 4, 2008 from http://www.masterteacherprogram.com/resources/notes_learning_styles.html

Illinois Online Network (ION). (2007). Retrieved February 25, 2008 from http://www.ion.uillinois.edu

Johnson, S. & Aragon, S. (2003). An instructional strategy framework for online learning environments. *New Directions for Adult and Continuing Education, 100*, 31–43.

Jonassen, D.H., Peck, K.L., Wilson, B.G. & Pfeiffer, W.S. (1998). Learning with technology: A constructivist perspective. New Jersey: Prentice Hall. Illinois.

Jung, I., Choi, S., Lim, C., & Leem, J. (2002). Effects of different types of interaction on learning achievement, satisfaction and participation in Web-based instruction. *Innovations in Education and Teaching International, 39*(2), 153–162.

Knowles, M. (1970). *The modern practice of adult education: Andragogy versus pedagogy.* New York: The Association Press.

Meacham, M. (2003). Using multiple intelligence theory in the virtual classroom. Retrieved on February 28, 2008 from http://www.learningcircuits.org/2003/jun2003/elearn.html

Moore, M., (1993). Transactional distance theory in D. Keegan (ed.). *Theoretical principles of distance education.* New York: Routledge.

National Education Association (n.d.). Guide to teaching with technology. Retrieved on February 22, 2008 from http://www.nea.org/technology/images/onlineteachguide.pdf

Pelz, B. (2004). (My) three principles of effective online pedagogy. *Journal of Asynchronous Learning Networks, 8*(3).

Shannon, S. (2003). Adult learning and CME. *The Lancet, 361*(9353), 266.

University of Maryland University College (n.d.). How do I learn? Retrieved on February 23, 2008 from http://www.umuc.edu/distance/de_orien/faqlearn.shtml

Vygotsky, L. (1978). *Mind in society: The development of higher psychological processes.* MA: Harvard University Press.

3 Infrastructure Considerations for Online Learning: Student, Faculty, and Technical Support

CHERYL A. FISHER

The growth in broadband, mobile technology and adaptive multimedia is both shifting and enhancing the experiences for distance learners. The available combinations of innovative pedagogic strategies have provided and encouraged novel learning technologies (Wade, 2007). However, the challenge remains to provide stimulating learning environments supported by technology.

The technical infrastructure necessary to support distance learning is critical when planning distance programs and includes a conglomeration of policies, services, and resources designated to support distance-learning efforts. Although distance learning is becoming more and more mainstream, not all academic institutions have a ubiquitous infrastructure in place to support the effort. Building infrastructure is dependent on institutional issues, technological issues, student support services, and faculty support. This chapter will address major factors and trends that are impacting academic institutions and distance education programs within the broad scope of the supporting infrastructure.

INSTITUTIONAL CONSIDERATIONS

Oftentimes the institution's mission and strategic plan is a good place to start looking for evidence of technology support for online learning. It is often these documents that will serve as the drivers for a technical infrastructure that is going to support distance-learning programs.

Pennsylvania State University (http://www.psu.edu/), a longstanding leader in distance education, developed guiding principles for infrastructure to support distance education, and they are based on policy, a dynamic programmatic mission, student and faculty support, and the need for policy change to support distance education efforts. Pennsylvania State University maintains that distance education is best recognized as an integrated part of the collegewide strategic goals and not as a separate activity.

When comparing strategic plans amongst similar large universities, several commonalities can be noted. These common elements include:

- An inclusive planning process with broad-based constituency involvement,
- A clear statement of the institution's mission and its aspirations for its current planning period,
- Comprehensive goals directly traceable to attainment of these aspirations and advancement of the institution's mission, and
- Clearly defined outcomes to assess the plan's success against nationally accepted measures.

What is evident is that a technical infrastructure is not directly mentioned in the common elements; however, these elements within the plans cannot be obtained without the ability to reach a broad-based constituency. To do this successfully, the institution should have a Web presence and outcome measures that utilize strong data-based management and networking capability.

Within nursing, the American Association of Colleges of Nursing (AACN, 1999) identifies factors that need to be addressed by nurses and other leaders in education and health care institutions, as well as external funders and policy makers, in order to take full advantage of the benefits of technology-supported education. These factors include:

- Superior distance education programs require substantial institutional financial investment in equipment, infrastructure, and faculty development.
- Local, regional, and national planning for multisite communications needs to consider coordination of services, compatibility and progressive upgrading of hardware, as well as policies that lower transmission costs within and across state lines.
- The use of distance technology, and Web-based media in particular, has raised questions regarding intellectual property and copyrights, privacy of educational dialogue, and other related legal and ethical issues that require continued clarification.
- Technology-mediated teaching strategies can dramatically change the way teaching and learning occur, challenging the traditional relationship of students to academic institutions. These strategies may change conventional thinking about how the quality of educational programs is assessed and what is required to support student learning (e.g., library access, counseling services, computing equipment, tuition, and financial aid).
- Nursing schools that use distance education technology have an advantage in recruiting students, and nursing schools are competing for students in their distance programs.

With supporting documents and other elements in place, an institution can better assess and plan where to focus resources and efforts necessary for a successful online program infrastructure. A recent review of institutional strategic plans conducted by Tallent-Runnels, Thomas, Lan, Cooper, Ahern, Shaw, and Liu (2006) revealed that few universities have policies, guidelines, or technical support for faculty members or students.

The American Distance Education Consortium (ADEC, 2008) states in their strategic plan that their purpose is to leverage active collaboration for advancing access to learner-centered educational programs anywhere in the world at any time. As a collaborative partner with Alfred P. Sloan Foundation, National Association of State Universities and Land Grant Colleges (NASULGC), and several government agencies (National Science Foundation, The U.S. Department of Agriculture, the National Agriculture Library and others), the ADEC sets forth goals that specify support to empower visionary thinking about education and technology. These goals are centered on collaboration of people, environments, hardware and connectivity, and software-driven tools that encourage and enhance teaching and learning specifically to engage people in the learning environment. Specific strategic initiatives in support of the ADEC goals include attention to:

- Global Science and Education Programs
- Disaster Relief and Homeland Security
- Innovation: Research and Development
- Human Capacity: Workforce Development and Commonwealth of Courses
- Digital Infrastructure

These initiatives address key issues, including global reach, research, and workforce development, all of which are critical elements for successful program development and expansion.

When making decisions about the digital infrastructure, it is sometimes easier to choose an available solution than it is to decide what solution is the best fit. It is critical to personalize and customize these services while understanding systems that are currently in place. It is important to understand that no system is going to provide all services required but interfaces may be the solution at hand.

INFORMATION TECHNOLOGY

When addressing technological issues for distance learning, the ADEC recommends that institutions establish appropriate technical requirements. This requires that compatibility needs be met, technology at origination and reception sites assure quality, that learners and facilitators be supported in their use of these technologies, and collaboration efforts be explored. It is becoming increasingly common to find institutional settings seeking external collaboration opportunities in order to share resources to meet these requirements.

Collaboration, consortia, and other alliances allow campuses to contribute content and resources to specific courses or areas of study in order to make most efficient use of time and money. The Connecticut Distance Learning Consortium (2007) is one example in which a collaborative eTutoring program has been created to meet the online tutoring needs of 34 participating two-year, and four-year public and private institutions of higher education. This inter-institutional program operates via a collaborative process that facilitates the sharing of tutors, organized on one schedule and one platform, which is accessed by all institutions. In addition, the collaboration between schools enables ongoing development of effective best practices protocols, as well as the design and delivery of an online tutoring platform that enables both synchronous and asynchronous tutoring opportunities.

The Western Interstate Commission for Higher Education (WICHE, 2008) was adopted in the 1950s by the western states to promote resource sharing, collaboration, and cooperative planning among their higher education systems. This collaboration seeks to improve access to higher education and to insure student success. Now a system with 15 states, members share program resources, information, technical expertise, services, and equipment related to distance learning.

Similarly, Iowa Communications Network (2008) invests in educational telecommunications and technology to support two-way interactive video conferencing in support of distance learning. The Iowa Communications Network is the country's premier fiber-optic network, committed to continued enhancement of distance learning. It provides Iowans with convenient access to education. The network makes it possible for remote and physically separated Iowans to interact in an efficient and cost effective manner, utilizing partnerships with education, medicine, and government agencies. As of 2008, this network was providing video to 750 classrooms around Iowa in schools, hospitals, libraries, and state government offices (Gillispie, Cassis, Jujinaka, McMahon, 2008).

Student Support Services

Online distance learners require multiple layers of support. Support services are critical to the success for the course and for the retention of online distance learners (Smith & Curry, 2005). These services include administrative support, technical support, mentor support, and other services.

Administrative support is often required in several forms, including: admissions, finance, registration, advising, and extension or deferral requests. It is imperative that these services be available and user friendly and that the administrative personnel responsible for these services be adequately trained in providing these services.

Counseling services need to be available to distance students and can be provided via synchronous or asynchronous means (chat room or e-mail) or by telephone. Student counseling centers often educate through informational pamphlets on various topics. The commercially available options are limited to specialized topics relevant to students. A counseling center can produce its own pamphlets; however, that would otherwise be costly and time consuming. An innovative alternative is the sharing of virtual pamphlets on the Web and providing links for counseling topics. However, human resources are necessary to evaluate and manage such resources to determine that they are appropriate and up to date.

The National Academic Advising Association Technology in Advising Commission (NACADA, 2008) suggests that distance students should have the same advising and counseling resources available to them that the other students have. These include workshops or training in the use of distance education technologies as required for students enrolled in courses or programs; access to the appropriate learning resources as required of distance learning students (i.e., basic skills, course tutorials, disability support, library services, and so forth); accurate information on the assumptions about the technical competence and skill level required; accurate and timely information, and an internal distance-learner network that connects all processes required of the distance learners and provides them with one point of contact for the services.

The NACADA Web site (http://www.nacada.ksu.edu) also lists academic advising resources available on the Internet, including topics ranging from career counseling to study skills, as well as multiple listing of academic advising Web page links to universities across the country. The core values described by NACADA reflect the fact that advisement is a personal process and establishes a relationship between the students and their institutions. Further, when done correctly, advisement is not just between the student and the advisor, but involves a team effort that includes the student support services of the institution, the student, and the advisor. According to the WICHE and NACADA, guidelines for developing an advisor's Web page (Carnevale, 2000), the basis for a comprehensive advising site should include the following elements:

1. *A clear and concise explanation of core curriculum (or general education) requirements.* Advisement usually involves a comprehensive explanation of curriculum requirements and a review of what a student has left to complete. Making this information available online will free up some time, will give students greater control and responsibility for the advisement process, and is essential information for students trying to determine course selection if they are unable to meet with an advisor.

2. *A Frequently Asked Questions (FAQ) section.* Every advisor spends a portion of the day repeating answers to the same questions. Putting answers to FAQs online saves time for staff and gives students access to answers as needed.

3. *Informational pages for special populations and self help assistance.* While there are certain common needs among students, there are segments of the population with additional unique concerns. Freshmen, students without declared majors, students on academic probation, and commuters are examples of groups with additional needs for support. Examples of information to include for advisement include

career or major information, study-skills-building worksheets, an explanation of the academic standing policy, information on how to get computer access and technical support, and parking information should onsite visits be necessary.

4. *Links to related university sites.* Holistic advisement involves supporting a student both academically and personally. Links to campus services such as student activities' calendars, campus organization pages, career services, academic lab locations and hours, and intramural offerings are needed to make sure all needs are being met.

5. *One-on-one access to advisors.* To generate a more personal environment and provide opportunities for interaction, advisors are experimenting with various forms of electronic communications. This is the most critical element in a comprehensive advising Web site. If advising were simply a matter of giving students a standardized package of information, there would be no reason to have advisors. Access to a qualified advisor can be achieved through the use of chat rooms, listservs, and emails, to mention a few of the most common methods.

WICHE (2001) evaluated online student support offerings at 15 colleges and universities and selected what they identified as best practices for integrating technology into student support services. The services evaluated a range from advisement and personal counseling to registration and financial aid. In 2003, WICHE went on to develop a "Cheat Sheet" to help organizations with general directions for developing online student services. These steps include:

1. Form a vision team and develop your campus's vision for student services online.
2. Determine initial student service focus and assemble a project design and development team.
3. Create a glossary of terms for student services and define the scope, budget, and timeline.
4. Write scenarios and record ARIs (assumptions, requirements, and issues).

5. Identify affected policies and take steps to address them.
6. Buy, build, or partner in the development of a technology solution to support plans for new service(s).
7. Test the new service with a pilot group of students.
8. Form an implementation team and develop an implementation plan.
9. Deploy your new service(s), gaining a yield of integrated IT systems, simple procedures, and online services.
10. Keep your institution happy with well-served students, faculty, staff, and others by upgrading the service(s) on an ongoing basis to maintain state-of-the-art services.

INFORMATION FOR PROSPECTIVE STUDENTS

The services recommended should begin with the first encounter that students are likely to have with a university when looking for an online course or program. The university home page should include information for students to help them decide if this is the right place for them. Recommendations for information include clear and highly visible information about online programs with direct links to more in-depth information. A personal readiness assessment (e.g., http://distance.wsu.edu/prospective/DDPquiz. asp) can help students determine if they are ready for online learning. This type of self-assessment can help determine how distance education will fit students' individual needs and reinforce the requirements of commitment and independent work in online environments.

Other helpful information to assess distance learning requirements can be found at the Jones College Web site (http://www.jones.edu/online-learning/requirements/). This site includes information on student learning requirements, system requirements, necessary computer skills, and contact information to help students decide if this is the best option for them.

Although these tools do not provide assurance of success, they help students identify technical skills and learning styles that will help them be successful online learners. A hardware and software assessment should be provided to students so they can determine the specifications necessary to participate in a course. A list of hardware, software, Internet service provider, e-mail, and browser requirements should be specified with definitions of terms included. A FAQ page is also often helpful, along with contact information such as e-mail or phone numbers for students to get additional information.

Admissions

The admissions process should be clearly delineated with specific steps for each part of the process. Admission requirements should be identified, and program-specific criteria would help students decide if they, in fact, want to apply. Methods for obtaining and submitting an application, deadlines, application tracking, and multiple payment methods are also recommended.

Another early step in the process that students should consider is a computer self-assessment. Many universities offering online education have these assessments available on the home page of their Web site. These assessments usually cover basic skills in Windows®, e-mail, hardware, and software.

Advising

NACADA states that providers of distance education programs must offer a minimum set of core services that assist distance learners in identifying and achieving their education goals. To facilitate this goal attainment, the following standards have been developed to address many categories as identified in the Academic Advising CAS Standards. These standards have been divided into three main categories: institutional, faculty advisor standards, and student standards. NACADA suggests the following standards for faculty advisors:

- A distance education program must provide for appropriate, real-time or delayed interaction between faculty, advisors, and students, and among students.
- The program provides faculty and advisors support to assist students in making informed choices about career

and academic goals, self-assessment, decision making, and evaluation of academic career options.

- The program provides faculty and advisors with the support to orient students to the distance-learning environment.
- The institution provides an environment in which faculty as advisors can work toward achieving competencies needed to be an advisor of distance learners (Thach & Murphy, 1995).

Although advising is critical for all students, it is even more essential that distance students feel they have a connection to someone at the institution. As these guidelines recommend, if students are to be successful, they need more than just quality courses online.

Content and learning support are also important to distance learning programs and may require services from tutors, writing centers, or campus libraries. The Western Cooperative for Telecommunications Education (2008) created a guide for developing distance-student services. These guidelines discuss tips for developing these services in addition to a discussion on the range of services that should be included and guidelines for best practices in delivering these services online. Although universities have increasingly recognized the value and need to provide online courses and programs, they often need help envisioning what services to provide and how to design them. The services addressed in this guide for students were determined to be "good practices" based on interactive Web services or for-profit companies that market software to support student needs. The student support services identified include:

- Information for prospective students
- Admissions
- Financial aid
- Registration
- Orientation services
- Academic advising
- Technical support
- Career services
- Library services
- Services for students with disabilities

- Personal counseling
- Instructional support and counseling
- Bookstore
- Services to promote a sense of community

The WICHE Web site lists multiple examples of online university student services sites.

FINANCIAL AID

Financial aid is a critical factor for students in the educational choices that they make. The issue of financial aid has an impact on course load, institutional choice, and whether the student can pursue higher education. Because of its importance, students should be able to easily access all financial aid information and forms directly from the Web. The information should include general information about financial aid, types of aid, details of cost, and the application process. The institution's financial aid policies should be disclosed for students in addition to federal school codes for the federal financial aid application. Dates, deadlines for application, and links to related sites are also important information sources and include general information for students.

REGISTRATION

Registration for online students is probably one of the most important online services that must be available and user friendly. This service will be used when students are registering for a program and each time they register for a course. Good practice recommendations include a full description of the registration process, identification of all registration method options available, relevant policies, an online scheduler, and online registration forms with clear instructions. It is important to note that many institutions have developed highly effective touch-tone registration systems, which may also serve distance students' needs.

Software for online student registration is increasingly available and easier to use, with increasing ability to meet student and higher education demands. Multiple systems are now available, providing features such as student registration, data-based course management, credit card payment capability, and custom report writing, just to mention a few. Additional features include financial aid application capability, records and registration, and the billing system. PeopleSoft, Zenegrade Corp, eClass Trak and Aceware are some examples of software available for course management described as a suite of products designed to meet the needs of higher educational institutions. This software manages institutional resources, student information, financial information, and human resources, among others. Various components can be used for faculty, students, advisors, and employees. These Web-based systems have the ability to be accessed anytime, anywhere in response to calls for flexibility of support services.

LIBRARY SERVICES

Within this constellation of support services, the library is also considered one of the most important academic units for online availability. The Association of College and Research Libraries' (ACRL, 2004) "Guidelines for Distance Learning Library Services" calls for a librarian or library administrator to plan, implement, coordinate, and evaluate library resources and services to address the information and skill needs of distance students. The guidelines further state in this document that traditional on-campus library services themselves cannot be stretched to meet the library needs of distance-learning students and faculty who face distinct and different challenges involving library access and information delivery.

The ACRL calls for resources and services in institutions of higher education to meet the needs of faculty, students, and academic support personnel, regardless of where they are located. Special funding, proactive planning, and promotion are necessary to deliver equivalent library services to achieve equivalent results in teaching and learning, and generally to maintain quality in distance learning programs.

Reasons cited to expand the "guidelines" have stemmed from the trend of nontraditional study rapidly becoming a major element in higher education, an increase in the diversity of educational opportunities, an increase in the number of unique environments where educational opportunities are offered, an increased recognition for the need for library services, and the requirement for services at locations other than main campuses (ACLR, 2004). Oftentimes it is the classroom that may have greater needs for library services. With the increase in technological innovation in the transmittal of information, a shift has been created towards an all-electronic university.

The library services recommended should be designed to effectively provide a wide range of information services and to be responsive to user needs. According to the ACRL, the following services, though not exhaustive, are essential:

1. Reference assistance
2. Computer-based bibliographic and informational services
3. Reliable, rapid, secure access to institutional and other networks, including the Internet
4. A program of library user instruction designed to instill independent and effective information literacy skills while specifically meeting the learner-support needs of the distance-learning community
5. Assistance with and instruction in the use of nonprint media and equipment
6. Reciprocal or contractual borrowing, or interlibrary loan services using broadest application of fair use of copyrighted materials
7. Prompt document delivery such as a courier system or electronic transmission
8. Access to reserve materials in accordance with copyright fair use policies
9. Adequate service hours for optimum access by users and consultative services
10. Promotion of library services to the distance learning community, including documented and updated policies, regulations, and procedures for systematic development and management of information resources.

As demand for electronic delivery of these services increases, demand for additional texts, journals, and other resources have also increased.

FACULTY SUPPORT AND WORKLOAD

Faculty support is another major consideration that institutions need to consider when developing distance programs. The time, knowledge, and skills that are required to design, develop, and teach online cannot be taken for granted or assumed by administrators to be basic faculty skills.

Faculty training for distance education has not traditionally been addressed by university settings, but it is becoming more widely recognized that teaching online is different from teaching in the classroom. As the value and complexity of this endeavor is realized, more institutions are investing time and resources into faculty training. The Indiana Higher Education Telecommunication System (IHETS, 2006) recommends that institutions engaged in the delivery of distance learning experiences provide appropriate training experiences for their faculty. IHETS suggests that faculty be exposed to various pedagogical strategies that are well suited to the distance-learning environment, and that exposure to in-services, workshops, and interactions with experienced peers be provided. Oftentimes this training is now being offered online.

IHETS identified the following principle and subprinciples relevant to faculty development. The main principle is that it is important for faculty who are engaged in the delivery of distance learning courses to take advantage of appropriate professional developmental experiences. The subprinciples include:

1. The faculty will seek out and participate in opportunities that expose them to various pedagogical strategies that are well suited to the distance-learning environment. This exposure could come from participation in in-services and workshops.

2. Faculty will seek out opportunities for collaborations and other interactions with faculty that have had success in the distance-learning environment. Those faculty members who have had success in distance learning should take a mentorship role with those who are seeking assistance.

3. The faculty will participate in the evaluation and selection of the software products that are going to be used for course development. The faculty should seek out and participate in ongoing training and technical support for various distance-learning development and delivery tools.

4. Faculty will understand the implications of teaching via distance, for example, the unique challenges presented by the various technologies.

5. The faculty will understand and observe the institution's policies regarding intellectual property and copyright.

These principles put the responsibility for course design and online facilitation on the faculty teaching the course. Ideally, faculty support for course development should include technical support, assurance of basic technical skills required to offer online courses, and available resources for support. For example, Penn State offers an online course titled, "Faculty Development 101" (http://www.worldcampus.psu.edu/AboutUs_FacultyDev101.shtml). The goals for this course provide faculty with an understanding of the issues involved in authoring or teaching an online course, an understanding of the support services available, and an understanding of the experiences of the distance student. This course serves as an excellent example of online faculty development that faculty can complete in their own time.

Faculty workload is a key factor that must be considered and defined. "Faculty workload" is defined as how much a faculty member teaches and how much of his or her work time is taken up with research, administration, and other duties. IHETS (2006) recommends a system of faculty incentives and rewards be developed cooperatively by faculty and the administration that encourages effort and recognizes achievement associated with the development and delivery of distance-learning courses. Additional recommendations include a mechanism for determining whether distance-learning course development and delivery will be included as part of a faculty member's workload or assigned on an overload basis. The evaluation process according to IHETS should be in accordance with institutional policy for teaching face-to-face courses.

Intellectual property and copyright law issues arise around who owns an electronic course or source materials once it is created. Does it belong to the institution, faculty member, or both? Historically, universities have given copyrights to faculty, allowing them to do as they wish with materials falling under copyright. However, when a faculty member develops a new invention or process, most campuses defined this creative contribution under their patent policies, because the institution had to commit a significant set of resources, and thus there was a sharing of any benefits derived from this intellectual property. Similarly, institutions could claim that when a course is developed using the university's software and university resources, significant institutional resources have been invested, thereby creating shared property. Dennis Thompson (1999) claims in his article, "Intellectual Property Meets Information Technology," that neither copyright nor patent policy is well suited to dealing with distributed learning materials. He argues that campuses have not defined adequate policies or reached a clear understanding of the issues around intellectual property, conflict of interest, and revenue sharing.

Faculty should also be provided with information regarding copyright laws and course content development for distance learning courses. Just because something is on the Web does not mean that it is there for the taking. The principle recommended by IHETS for determining copyright law compliance is that content developed for distance learning courses will comply with copyright law. The subprinciples include:

1. The process recommended for determining copyright law compliance is as follows:
   - Attention will be paid to the rights and privileges regarding transmission of materials as defined in Section 110(2) of the U.S. Copyright Law (See Appendix A).

- If Section 110(2) does not apply, "fair use," as defined in Section 107 (See Appendix), may apply. The nature and amount of the work used, and the purpose and effect of the use will be weighed to determine if fair use applies.
- If the planned use of a copyrighted work cannot be addressed by Section 110(2) or Section 107, permission of the content owner may be required.

2. Be aware how to obtain copyright permission. Some institutions may provide assistance in obtaining such permission.

In summary, the importance of institutional commitment from the strategic plan to the home page must be evidenced by faculty support and a complex technological structure. There clearly needs to be a commitment on the part of the institution, the faculty, and the students themselves in order to have a well-supported distance program. When considering recommended guidelines and the multiple systems and resources mentioned throughout this chapter, an organization's strategic plan can help to support the requirements for establishment, maintenance, and growth of a distance program.

REFERENCES

American Distance Education Consortium (ADEC). (2008). ADEC Strategic Plan. Retrieved April 18, 2008, from http://www.adec.edu/admin/papers/distance-learning_principles.html

Association of College and Research Libraries (ACRL). (2004). Standards and Guidelines. Retrieved April 18, 2008, from http://www.ala.org/acrl/guides/distlrng.html

American Association of Colleges of Nursing (1999). AACN White Paper: Distance technology in nursing education. Retrieved April 26, 2008, from http://www.aacn.nche.edu/Publications/WhitePapers/whitepaper.htm

Carnevale, D. (2000). Commission's Web site helps colleges put student services online. *The Chronicle of Higher Education.* Retrieved April 26, 2008, from, http://chronicle.com

Connecticut Distance Learning Consortium. (n.d.). Retrieved April 22, 2008 at http://www.ctdlc.org

Gillispie, J., Cassis, J., Jujinaka, T., & McMahon, G. (2008). Meeting the shifting perspective: The Iowa Communications Network. *Distance Learning,* 5(1), 1–11.

Indiana Higher Education Telecommunication System. (2006). Retrieved April 18, 2008, from http://www.ihets.org/progserv/networking/itn

Iowa Communications Network (2008). Retrieved April 26, 2008, from http://www.icn.state.ia.us

National Academic Advising Association Technology in Advising Commission (NACADA). (2008). Retrieved April 21, 2008, from http://www.psu.edu/dus/ncta/linkacad.htm

National Academic Advising Association (2008). Retrieved April 26, 2008, from http://www.nacada.ksu.edu

Pennsylvania State University (2008). Retrieved April 26, 2008, from http http://psu.edu

Pennsylvania State World Campus (2008). Retrieved April 26, 2008, from (http://www.worldcampus.psu.edu/AboutUs_FacultyDev101.shtml).

Smith, L. & Curry, M. (2005). Twelve tips for authoring on-line distance learning medical post registration programs. *Medical Teacher, 27*(4), 316–324.

Tallent, M., Thomas, J., & Cooper L. (2006). Teaching courses online: A review of the research. *Review of Educational Research, 76*(1), 93–135.

Wade, V. & Ashman, H. (2007). Evolving the infrastructure for distance learners. *IEE Computer Society.* Retrieved April 26, 2008, from http://csdl2.computer.org/comp/mags/ic/2007/03/w3016.pdf

Western Interstate Commission for Higher Education. (2008). Retrieved April, 26, 2008, from http://www.wiche.edu

Western Cooperative for Telecommunications Education. (2008). Retrieved April 26, 2008, from http://www.wcet.info/about

Thach E. & Murphy, K. (1995). Competencies for distance education professionals. *Educational Technology Research and Development, 43*(1), 57–79.

Thompson, D. (1999). Intellectual property meets information technology, *Educom Review, 34*(2), 14–21.

APPENDIX A

110. Limitations on exclusive rights: Exemption of certain performances and displays

Notwithstanding the provisions of section 106, the following are not infringements of copyright: (2) except with respect to a work produced or marketed primarily for performance or display as part of mediated instructional activities transmitted via digital networks, or a performance or display that is given by means of a copy or phonorecord that is not lawfully made and acquired under this title, and the transmitting government body or accredited nonprofit educational institution knew or had reason to believe was not lawfully made and acquired, the performance of a nondramatic literary or musical work or reasonable and limited portions of any other work, or display of a work in an amount comparable to that which is typically displayed in the course of a live classroom session, by or in the course of a transmission, if—

A the performance or display is made by, at the direction of, or under the actual supervision of an instructor as an integral part of a class session offered as a regular part of the systematic mediated instructional activities of a governmental body or an accredited nonprofit educational institution;

B the performance or display is directly related and of material assistance to the teaching content of the transmission;

C the transmission is made solely for, and, to the extent technologically feasible, the reception of such transmission is limited to—

   i students officially enrolled in the course for which the transmission is made; or

   ii officers or employees of governmental bodies as a part of their official duties or employment; and

D the transmitting body or institution—

   i institutes policies regarding copyright, provides informational materials to faculty, students, and relevant staff members that accurately describe, and promote compliance with, the laws of the United States relating to copyright, and provides notice to students that materials used in connection with the course may be subject to copyright protection; and

ii in the case of digital transmissions—

I applies technological measures that reasonably prevent—

aa retention of the work in accessible form by recipients of the transmission from the transmitting body or institution for longer than the class session; and

bb unauthorized further dissemination of the work in accessible form by such recipients to others; and

II does not engage in conduct that could reasonably be expected to interfere with technological measures used by copyright owners to prevent such retention or unauthorized further dissemination;

In paragraph (2), the term "mediated instructional activities" with respect to the performance or display of a work by digital transmission under this section refers to activities that use such work as an integral part of the class experience, controlled by or under the actual supervision of the instructor and analogous to the type of performance or display that would take place in a live classroom setting. The term does not refer to activities that use, in 1 or more class sessions of a single course, such works as textbooks, course packs, or other material in any media, copies or phonorecords of which are typically purchased or acquired by the students in higher education for their independent use and retention or are typically purchased or acquired for elementary and secondary students for their possession and independent use. For purposes of paragraph (2), accreditation—

A with respect to an institution providing post-secondary education, shall be as determined by a regional or national accrediting agency recognized by the Council on Higher Education Accreditation or the United States Department of Education; and

B with respect to an institution providing elementary or secondary education, shall be as recognized by the applicable state certification or licensing procedures.

For purposes of paragraph (2), no governmental body or accredited nonprofit educational institution shall be liable for infringement by reason of the transient or temporary storage of material carried out through the automatic technical process of a digital transmission of the performance or display of that material as authorized under paragraph (2). No such material stored on the system or network controlled or operated by the transmitting body or institution under this paragraph shall be maintained on such system or network in a manner ordinarily accessible to anyone other than anticipated recipients. No such copy shall be maintained on the system or network in a manner ordinarily accessible to such anticipated recipients for a longer period than is reasonably necessary to facilitate the transmissions for which it was made.

LIMITATIONS ON EXCLUSIVE RIGHTS: FAIR USE

Notwithstanding the provisions of sections 106 and 106A, the fair use of a copyrighted work, including such use by reproduction in copies or phonorecords or by any other means specified by that section, for purposes such as criticism, comment, news reporting, teaching (including multiple copies for classroom use), scholarship, or research, is not an infringement of copyright. In determining whether the use made of a work in any particular case is a fair use the factors to be considered shall include:

1. the purpose and character of the use, including whether such use is of a commercial nature or is for nonprofit educational purposes;
2. the nature of the copyrighted work;
3. the amount and substantiality of the portion used in relation to the copyrighted work as a whole; and
4. the effect of the use upon the potential market for or value of the copyrighted work.

The fact that a work is unpublished shall not itself bar a finding of fair use if such finding is made upon consideration of all the above factors.

4

Technologies and Competencies Needed for Online Learning

SUSAN K. NEWBOLD AND CHERYL A. FISHER

Nursing schools may employ any of the numerous course management systems available to create online learning environments and supplement those systems with technologies that will enrich the learning experience and customize them to fit their particular demographic. This chapter will investigate the features of course management systems and the technology that will support online learning. In addition, the competencies needed to be successful in online learning environments will be discussed.

Distance education implies a separation between the student and the teacher. With the least complex arrangement, distance education in nursing can take the form of a correspondence course, where written communication is the only interaction between the student and the teacher. At the most complex configuration, it is possible to enroll in a series of courses leading to a degree and never enter the campus or meet the instructors face-to-face. Courses can be self-paced (individuals moving through the courses at their own pace) or cohort (a group moving at the same pace).

Course management systems are Web-based systems that support academic learning. Carliner (2005) outlines activities that are available to faculty in course management systems. They are able to do the following:

- Create course material that can be placed in the system;
- Track student quizzes, exam grades, and assignments through a grade book and student participation through course statistics;
- Offer students different venues (e.g., chat rooms, discussion boards) to discuss course content;
- Communicate information about the course through announcements and virtual chat rooms.

Course management systems are easy to learn and allow faculty to easily create their courses. Some challenges are that the systems may have limited flexibility in design function, a limited capacity to provide interactive e-learning, limited testing and record keeping abilities, not to mention the increasing cost of the systems (Carliner, 2005).

Course delivery systems are selected with input from faculty and instructional designers. Prior to selecting a delivery system, the needs of the learners and the content of the courses should be determined. In some organizations, others will dictate the technology and in some cases the instructor is allowed to select the technology. There are many popular course management systems used in academic settings. Among the more popular are WebCT, Blackboard, and Moodle. Blackboard is a closed-source system, which means that the source codes of the program are locked and cannot be changed. Moodle is open-source system, which means that the software is free. The companies charge for service agreements, but these are voluntarily purchased. In an open-source system, the lines and codes that allow the system to function are visible. Therefore, the codes can be changed to better meet the needs of the schools using them. Perens (1999) describes three rights that are assured when using open source systems. They are:

- The right to make and distribute copies of the program.
- The right to have access to the software's source code.

■ The right to make improvements and changes to the program by changing the source code to meet the needs of the learners who will use the system.

Some schools have the expertise to develop their own online course delivery tools that can be tailored to the individual school. A school can either purchase the software for installation at the school or purchase the use of the software over the Internet. Course management systems have a core set of functionalities and have similar components:

1. Course communication features may include discussion board, chat, e-mail, and a collaborative whiteboard.
2. Course assessment can include tests of different kinds to be administered. Other assignments can be distributed, either at the beginning of the course or just before needed. Models of excellent work can be posted as exemplars to other students.
3. Course management through the use of an online grade book, course rosters, student access tracking, and student password information are the usual tools.
4. Course information such as the syllabus, instructor home page, calendar, course announcements, and task lists are also important features. The home page may include facilitator office hours (physical and virtual), course topics to be covered, textbook purchasing information, course objectives, and grading policies. A link to the facilitator e-mail and telephone number should be provided. Links to discussion groups and online forums that students can use to report problems or provide biographical information and a picture should be present. Materials in the classroom can be posted as Web pages or downloadable files (such as Microsoft® PowerPoint™ handouts). Reference material will include bibliographies and articles or perhaps a link to a virtual library.
5. Course didactic features include file uploading and downloading (for example moving Microsoft® PowerPoint™, Microsoft® Word™, Microsoft® Excel™ files), streaming video and audio, external Web links, and course module builders.

COMPARISON OF ONLINE DELIVERY SYSTEMS

When selecting a system, a determination should be made if software is used elsewhere on the campus. Technical support, maintenance, software fees, and so forth can be shared if the same system is purchased. If the School of Nursing is embarking upon the initial effort to find a system, first the assessment of needs must be conducted. Then the software is found that satisfies those needs, followed by the hardware that supports the software.

A table can be developed to compare the needs of the School of Nursing and the features of the online delivery systems. Some of the school's needs may be to create and grade essay tests or to support faculty in designing the learning space. Each school has different needs, and the needs determine what the school will require of the software package. When searching for an appropriate online delivery system, sources on the Web can be used to compare features of the various products. One site is EduTools (2008) (www.edutools. info), which offers a comparison of features for course management systems for the purpose of providing information decision-making. Twenty-five course management systems can be compared using the features outlined in Table 4.1. Compare the features of various course management systems to the list of your needs and gather information to make a decision about the system that will best meet your needs.

Software can be added on to course management systems to enhance the students' learning experiences. Three examples of these add-ons are: streaming media, e-Packs, and QuestionMark.

Streaming media is an information delivery method that "enables real-time or on-demand access to audio, video, and multimedia content via the Internet or an intranet" (Adobe Dynamic Media Group, 2001, p. 3). Streaming media features the following characteristics: enables real-time or on-demand access to audio, video, and multimedia content via the Internet or an intranet; enables the near real-time transmission of events recorded in video or audio, and is sometimes called "Live-Live" or Webcasting; can be conveniently distributed on-demand as prerecorded or pre-edited media that can be accessed anytime and anywhere (Adobe Dynamic Media Group, 2001). The streaming media advantages include: no waiting time for

Table 4.1

EDUTOOLS COMPARISON FEATURES (EDUTOOLS, 2008)

LEARNER TOOLS	SUPPORT TOOLS	TECHNICAL SPECIFICATIONS
Communication ■ Discussion Forums ■ Discussion Management ■ File Exchange ■ Internal email ■ Online Journal/notes ■ Real-time chat ■ Whiteboard	Administration Tools ■ Authentication ■ Course Authorization ■ Registration integration ■ Hosted Services	Hardware/Software ■ Client Browser Required ■ Database Requirements ■ UNIX Server ■ Windows Server
Productivity Tools ■ Bookmarks ■ Calendar/Progress Review ■ Searching within course ■ Work offline/synchronize ■ Orientation/help	Course Delivery Tools ■ Test types ■ Automated Testing Management ■ Automated Testing Support ■ Online Marking Tools ■ Online Grade Book ■ Course Management ■ Student Tracking	Company Details/Licensing ■ Company Profile ■ Costs/Licensing ■ Open Source ■ Optional extras
Student Involvement Tools ■ Group work ■ Community Networking ■ Student Portfolios	Content Development Tools ■ Accessibility Compliance ■ Content Sharing/reuse ■ Course templates ■ Customized look and feel ■ Instructional design Tools ■ Instructional Standards Compliance	

the media to download—the media is processed and played and then discarded so copyright concerns are reduced, and events can be witnessed in real time (Adobe Dynamic Media Group, 2001). An added feature is that the media can be downloaded and saved providing the content is proprietary to the course. Streaming media is an emerging technology that can bring exciting learning opportunities to the online classroom through the instructor sharing content with students and students using the technology to complete assignments.

E-Pack is publisher-provided content that can be uploaded into your course. E-Packs are "fast, easy, and flexible ways to deliver high-quality, media-rich online content" (Blackboard, 2004). Blackboard (2004) suggests that using e-Packs will save faculty time in developing their own course material while allowing faculty to customize the content, and they give students access to high-quality, media-rich content. E-Packs can be accessed on many topics and in many disciplines. The content is developed by higher education publishers such as McGraw-Hill and Thomson Learning.

QuestionMark is an example of an assessment management system that can be added to the course management system. QuestionMark allows the instructor to author questions, schedule assessments, deliver assessments, and analyze results through customized reports. The instructor can create secure question banks and exams with randomized questions, and students can obtain feedback as soon as they complete and submit the exam for grading. QuestionMark offers more diversity than the assessment packages that are within course management systems (QuestionMark, 2008).

Student Requirements

The student needs to have a computer with access to the Internet in order to participate in the course. Passwords are used in order to identify the student. Course management systems offer tutorials in order to help the student experience the various course features. Web sites are also available that can help students identify their readiness for taking a course online such as this one offered at Online Learning. net (http://www.onlinelearning.net/OLE/holwselfassess.html?s=029. b030z6841.0240528690).

The Maryland Online Web site offers tools for the student that include an assessment to determine if learning online is the best strategy for the student. This assessment can be found at http://www.marylandonline.org/assessments/tech_savvy. Maryland Online also lists the technical skills requirements for students, and these can be found at the same Web site. Schools with online programs should include an on-site orientation to online learning or a "virtual" orientation that is available on their Web site.

The nurse at all levels must have some expertise using information technology at the job site and in an educational setting. Both the course instructor and the student must have basic computer competencies in order to create, maintain, facilitate, and take an online course. Staggers, Gassert, and Curran (2001) studied minimal competencies that nurses must possess. They identify 31 competencies at the beginning nurse level, as well as fundamental information management and computer technology skills. Examples of these skills are as follows:

- Uses telecommunication devices (i.e., modem, other devices) to communicate with other systems (e.g., access data, upload, download);
- Uses e-mail (e.g., create, send, respond, use attachments);
- Uses presentation graphics (e.g., PowerPoint™) to create slides, displays;
- Uses multimedia presentations;
- Uses word processing;
- Demonstrates keyboarding (i.e., typing) skills;
- Uses spreadsheets;
- Uses networks to navigate systems (e.g., files servers, World Wide Web);
- Is able to navigate Windows (e.g., manipulate files using file manager, determine active printer, access installed applications, create and delete directories).

Instructor Competencies for Online Learning

Teaching in an online learning environment is different from teaching in the traditional classroom. The instructor has to overcome potential barriers caused by technology, time, and place to create an optimal environment for achieving educational goals. The instructor or facilitator must make sure the course is running smoothly and that barriers (they will certainly happen) are overcome quickly. It is important to make the technology as transparent as possible, and it should be viewed as a tool to enable learning the content of the course.

The instructor must be offered some level of training. For example, if an instructor has utilized Lotus Learning Space® and the school is changing platforms to WebCT®, perhaps only a written handout is needed pointing out the differences in the two software packages. The instructor must know some file management techniques and tips such as transferring files, adding attachments, word processing, initiating chats, finding a file in a hierarchical system, and printing files. It is helpful to be able to use spreadsheet and presentation software (like Microsoft® PowerPoint™), and to possess basic skills with database software, as well as know about basic security controls. The more the educator knows about the technical workings of the course management system, the more control he or she has over the course. The educator may elect to learn software tools for developing the home page such as HTML and Dreamweaver, or Microsoft® FrontPage. Protocols such as FTP ("file transfer protocol") can be used to upload and download files to and from the students.

In summary, a number of course management systems can be used to deliver quality online courses, and a variety of add-ons can be used to enhance the learning environment. These add-ons continue to offer faculty opportunities to enrich student learning experiences utilizing multimedia and assessment capabilities while responding to student preferences for course content delivery. With the competencies discussed in this chapter, students and instructors can take advantage of these technologies with minimal additional technical skills and creative pedagogical approaches to course design and delivery.

REFERENCES

Adobe Dynamic Media Group. (2001). A streaming media primer. Retrieved April 28, 2008, from http://www.adobe.com/products/aftereffects/pdfs/AdobeStr.pdf

Blackboard. Retrieved April 28, 2008, from: http://www.blackboard.com

Carliner, S. (2005). Course management systems versus learning management systems. *Learning Circuits.* Retrieved April 28, from http://www.learningcircuits.org/2005/nov2005/carliner.htm

EduTools. (2008). Providing decision-making tools for the EDU community. Retrieved April 28, 2008, from http://www.edutools.info/item_list.jsp?pj=4

Perens, B. (1999). Open Source Definition. Retrieved April 28, 2008, from http://www.oreilly.com/catalog/opensources/book/perens.html

QuestionMark. (2008). Retrieved April 28, 2008, from http://www.questionmark.com/us/perception/index.aspx

Staggers, N., Gassert, C. A., & Curran, C. (2001). Informatics competencies for nurses at four levels of practice. *Journal of Nursing Education,* 40(7), 303–316.

WebCT. Retrieved June 15, 2003, from http://www.webct.com

5

Reconceptualizing the Online Course

CAROL A. O'NEIL

The stage between making the decision to use online learning strategies and actually developing the learning environment is most important and pertinent. Reconceptualizing the learning material means going from, "Okay, I have this learning material," to using online pedagogy, infrastructure, and technology to make decisions about how the learning material will be presented online. Reconceptualizing is a series of if-then statements. It is a decision tree in which strengths, purpose, and resources are examined in order to make decisions about the best approach to use in presenting the learning material. Reconceptualizing is answering questions and using the answers to guide the development of online learning and communication environments.

The decision tree in Figure 5.1 will guide your decision making. The tree comprises questions, possible answers, and possible actions. These questions were developed using the "Guidelines for the Use of Distance Technology in Nursing Education," an appendix of the American Association of Colleges of Nursing (1999) White Paper; "Distance Technology in Nursing Education." Questions will

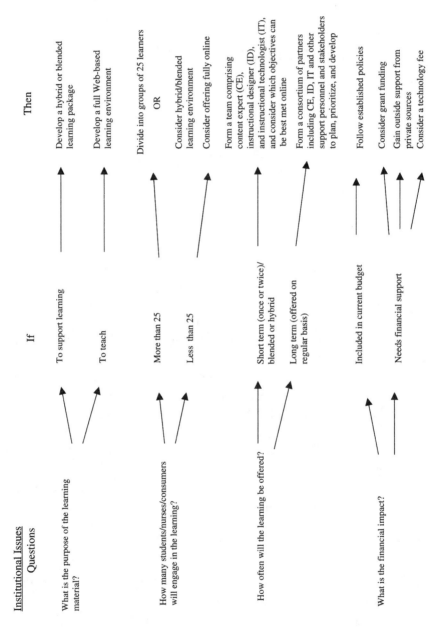

Figure 5.1. Decision tree to reconceptualize learning online.

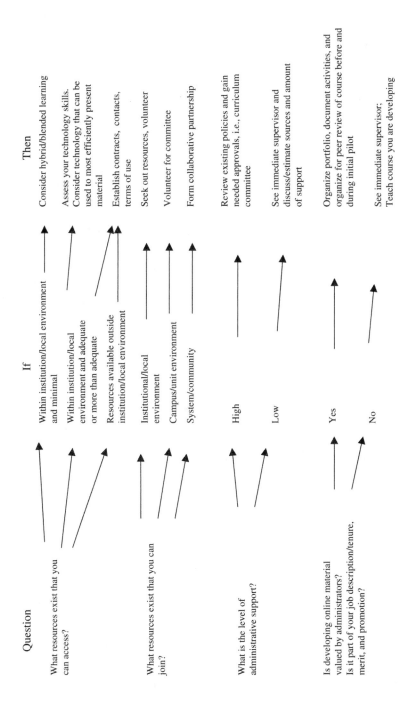

Question

What resources exist that you can access?

If

Within institution/local environment and minimal

Within institution/local environment and adequate or more than adequate

Resources available outside institution/local environment

Then

Consider hybrid/blended learning

Assess your technology skills. Consider technology that can be used to most efficiently present material

Establish contracts, contacts, terms of use

What resources exist that you can join?

Institutional/local environment

Campus/unit environment

System/community

Seek out resources, volunteer

Volunteer for committee

Form collaborative partnership

What is the level of administrative support?

High

Low

Review existing policies and gain needed approvals, i.e., curriculum committee

See immediate supervisor and discuss/estimate sources and amount of support

Is developing online material valued by administrators? Is it part of your job description/tenure, merit, and promotion?

Yes

No

Organize portfolio, document activities, and organize for peer review of course before and during initial pilot

See immediate supervisor; Teach course you are developing

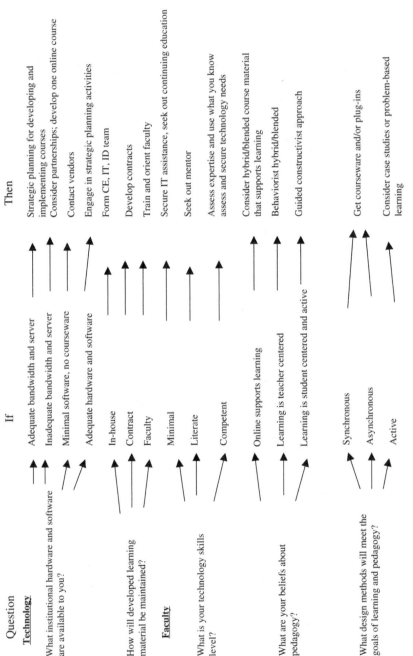

Question	If	Then
Technology		
What institutional hardware and software are available to you?	Adequate bandwidth and server	Strategic planning for developing and implementing courses
	Inadequate bandwidth and server	Consider partnerships; develop one online course
	Minimal software, no courseware	Contact vendors
	Adequate hardware and software	Engage in strategic planning activities
How will developed learning material be maintained?	In-house	Form CE, IT, ID team
	Contract	Develop contracts
	Faculty	Train and orient faculty
Faculty		
What is your technology skills level?	Minimal	Secure IT assistance, seek out continuing education
	Literate	Seek out mentor
	Competent	Assess expertise and use what you know assess and secure technology needs
What are your beliefs about pedagogy?	Online supports learning	Consider hybrid/blended course material that supports learning
	Learning is teacher centered	Behaviorist hybrid/blended
	Learning is student centered and active	Guided constructivist approach
What design methods will meet the goals of learning and pedagogy?	Synchronous	Get courseware and/or plug-ins
	Asynchronous	
	Active	Consider case studies or problem-based learning

Figure 5.1 (*continued*)

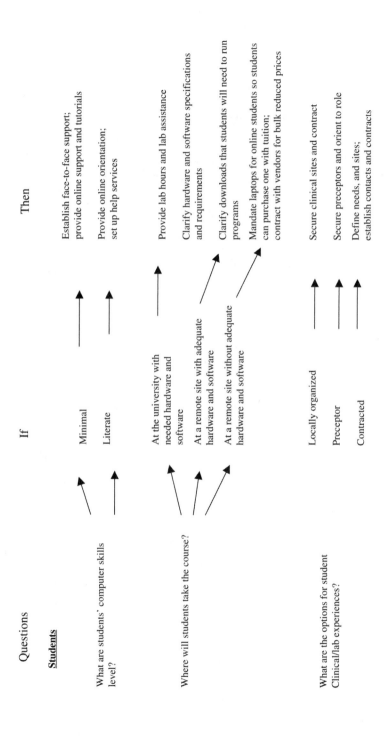

Questions

Students

What are students' computer skills level?

If

Minimal

Literate

Then

Establish face-to-face support; provide online support and tutorials

Provide online orientation; set up help services

Where will students take the course?

At the university with needed hardware and software

At a remote site with adequate hardware and software

At a remote site without adequate hardware and software

Provide lab hours and lab assistance

Clarify hardware and software specifications and requirements

Clarify downloads that students will need to run programs

Mandate laptops for online students so students can purchase one with tuition; contract with vendors for bulk reduced prices

What are the options for student Clinical/lab experiences?

Locally organized

Preceptor

Contracted

Secure clinical sites and contract

Secure preceptors and orient to role

Define needs, and sites; establish contacts and contracts

be posed about institutional issues, technology, faculty, and students. Possible answers to the questions are given, and action based on each of the possible answers is proposed.

USING THE DECISION TREE

The following is an example of how answering the decision tree questions can guide your decision making. A school of nursing is considering online courses. The dean meets with the department chair and a faculty member, Dr. G., who has experience in teaching online, to discuss the feasibility of moving the RN to BSN program online. The school has a strategic plan that includes online learning. The strategic plan was developed with input from faculty. This information about institutional factors leads to the conclusion that support for online programs is strong. The dean is willing to provide an information technology (IT) expert and instructional design (ID) support. The program will enroll more than 25 students and will be long term. The current budget will support development activities. No policies about online courses are available.

The school has its own server and enough bandwidth for a limited number of courses. One instructional designer is available for consultation, but no maintenance support personnel are available. The school has three-year-old desktop computers for faculty members. Microsoft Office® Web development software is available. Several laptops are available to faculty and all computers have Internet access. Computer laboratories are available for students, with over 50 terminals in the school of nursing.

Dr. G. has been involved in a project to guide and mentor faculty to teach online for a year. She is computer literate and is a content expert (CE) in community health nursing. She believes that students learn through interacting with learning material and that students can learn from each other. Dr. G. believes that faculty motivate and guide learning. She would like to provide a variety of learning options for students. Dr. G. would like to include course content, bulletin boards for discussions, small groups for students to complete activities, and synchronous chat rooms for office hours. She would like student assessment to include participation in discussions, assignments, and exam grades. Students should have computers available for use outside the school of nursing.

Decisions

Based on this information, one course in the RN to BSN program would be developed. This course would have a community focus, and Dr. G. would develop and teach it. Teaching the course would be included in her workload, and developing the course would be considered "service" and included as a "merit" activity. The current instructional designer would contract with a courseware vendor and would teach Dr. G. how to use the courseware. Dr. G. would partner with a technical person (IT) and the two would work as a CE and IT team. The course would be organized by modules. Each module would have objectives, readings, content, small-group activities, and large-group discussion questions. Content would be disseminated in written and audio formats. Grading would include projects, participation, and exams.

The course is marketed prior to and at course registration and students register in the usual way. The names of the registered students were sent to Dr. G., and she entered the students into her online course. While the pilot was in process, the faculty administrator for the undergraduate program, Dr. G., and the Instructional Designer met to plan for future courses. Evaluation information from the pilot course was solicited several times during the course and at the end of the course and was used to refine the course and to design other courses. One new course per faculty member was added each semester for a year. The lessons learned were shared with faculty who were developing their courses. The team guided and supported faculty developing and teaching new courses online. Faculty new to teaching online were invited to join the Web-Based Teaching Committee, and the team grew each semester. Sharing ideas and experiences with peers was essential for the development of the program. Through this group, policies, online student registration and support, and student and faculty support systems were developed.

Another possible scenario that might exist is high technical support and minimal faculty skill. If the faculty is motivated and willing to learn to develop online courses, go online. If there is moderate support and high resources, go online. If there is minimal support and resources, consider hybrid or blended courses and build support and stakeholders. A hybrid or blended course combines technology and traditional classroom strategies.

Developing a hybrid or blended course is an excellent way to begin while gathering resources, support, and experience. Gravitate toward a level at which the effort will be successful. Maximize the resources available and incorporate new resources and technology that will enhance your course. Pilot the material, have the material peer reviewed, and solicit learner feedback frequently for incorporation into course revisions.

RECONCEPTUALIZING COURSES

Hybrid or Blended Courses

The administration decides to put a portion of the course material online. This is called "blended learning," which is defined as augmenting traditional face-to-face learning with technology. It is the mixing of technology with activities and interaction to create a seamless transition between learning and working.

What are some options for blended learning? Look at the learning goals and objectives, the available technology, and the skill level of the faculty. Think about maximizing the use of technology to create the most effective environment for student learning. Some of the options are described below:

- Use voice, video, text, or any combination thereof to put the essential content online, so that you can use class time for discussion activities and case studies. For example, narrate some psychiatric or didactic nursing class lectures to create a mini-lecture using Microsoft PowerPoint® and RealPlayer®. Limit content to a specific unit of study, for example, depression.

Give essential knowledge on depression that will accomplish the objectives. The learning material should be limited to about twenty minutes. The required reading on depression and the mini-lecture on depression should be completed before class. Use in-class time for small group discussion of case studies. The case studies will help the student to begin to apply the content. Use the scenario of depression in a teenager, a postpartum woman, or an adult. Care plans can be the outcome of the case study.

- Use class time to impart content and use online environments to support learning through links relevant to the learning material.
- Use online support for administrative and organizational functions such as grading, computerized examinations, announcements, directions, and syllabus presentation. Use the online environment for discussion of case studies. Set up a discussion forum for each case study or divide the students into small groups to discuss the case study and develop care plans.

Mental Models

Once the decision to present the learning material online is made, the next step is to develop plans that will maximize the available resources, including hardware and software. It is more effective to use what is available to its optimal capacity and use what is known to the fullest potential to produce a learning environment that will maximize assets. The "lowest common denominator" should be attained, which means that not all students have access to the same hardware and software or bandwidth. If a course is built using software that the student does not have or does not have access to, the student will become frustrated and dissatisfied. For example, when using a mini-lecture requiring plug-ins for viewing multimedia or audio files, the content of this mini-lecture may not be available to students with older computers or slow dial-up connections. Providing content using links and text will provide information to a larger audience, because it is a lowest common denominator and the most accessible to students.

How can the course instructor convert traditional learning material to an online learning environment? What may be used to create the online learning environment? These are the next questions in reconceptualizing online learning environments. Because of the lack of visual feedback from students (shaking of heads while you are lecturing or closed eyes and bobbing heads), online learning environments need to give students a clear picture of what they are learning and how they will learn it. In the traditional classroom, the teacher begins a learning session by telling the students what they will learn (learning objectives), gives them the information needed to learn the content, and then the teacher summarizes what the students have learned. A traditional teacher begins by saying "Today we are going to learn about depression" and at the end might say, "Let me summarize what we have said about depression," so the student knows where they are in the learning process. In online learning environments, students still need to know where they are in the learning process and this is done through mental models. Mental models give meaning to concepts and promote the transfer of knowledge from the "didactic" to the "real" world.

Example of Reconceptualizing Online Learning Environments

Let us follow Dr. G. in the reconceptualization process. Dr. G. reconceptualized an undergraduate Community/Public Health Nursing course. She considered her pedagogical beliefs that students learn differently and have unique learning styles. She decided to include learning strategies such as text, verbal, and discussion modes of learning to accommodate a variety of learning styles. Dr. G. decided to organize by modules. The traditional classroom course was organized by "week"—Week 1, Week 2, and so forth. The online course includes objectives and readings, content, and small group activities. The content outline looks like this:

Community/Public Health Nursing

Module 1: History of Community/Public Health Nursing
- Objectives and Readings
- Content
- Activities

Module 2: Influences on the Practice of Community/Public Health Nursing
- Objectives and Readings
- Content
- Activities

Module 3: Cultural Influences on the Practice of Community/Public Health Nursing
- Objectives and Readings
- Content
- Activities

This organizing framework continued to Module 15 for a 15-week course. This design was cumbersome and needed streamlining. Dr. G. looked at the content and decided that the course really contained four areas of content: History and Scope, Practice, Focus, and Tools. Dr. G. shifted the modules into four content areas as illustrated in Figure 5.2.

Each section contains several of the original modules. History and Scope comprises modules 1, 2, and 3; Practice comprises modules 4, 5, 6, and 7; Focus comprises modules 8 and 9; Tools comprises modules 10, 11, and 12. The content areas and the modules within that area are presented in the same color and each content area has a different color. Each module contains objectives and readings, mini-lectures, and activities. This reconceptualization has several advantages. Students repeatedly see the four content

History and Scope	Focus
Practice	**Tools**

Figure 5.2 The reconceptualized course.

areas, and these become the four concepts of Community/Public Health Nursing. The concepts, called "mental models," are consistently reinforced when the student accesses the course content. Mental models give meaning to concepts and promote the transfer of knowledge from the "didactic" to the "real" world. When the student sees the word "Tools" over and over, the student forms a mental model that community/public health nursing has tools, and one of those tools is epidemiology (a module).

Operationalizing the mental model in an activity strengthens the impact of the mental model. For example, one of the activities in the "Tools" mental model could include a case study of an epidemic of influenza in a community.

Reconceptualizing a course provides students with a "map" of the course so they can see what the course is about, where they have been, and where they are going in the course.

Pedagogy

First consider the pedagogical beliefs and think about what can be used to operationalize those beliefs. Ask yourself the following questions:

- Do you prefer one learning style or many?
- Do you believe that group communication will support learning?
- Do you support synchronous communication?
- Do you support asynchronous communication?

Which technology will be used to create the course is the next question. Some options are audio, video, links, podcasts, wikis, text, or PowerPoint® presentations. Start with what is familiar and consider the preferred philosophy of teaching and learning.

Example of Reconceptualizing Pedagogy

Consider how Dr. G. operationalizes her philosophical and pedagogical beliefs about teaching and learning online. Dr. G. chose to include mini-lectures with voice synchronized PowerPoint®. The mini-lecture included content that was pertinent to meeting module objectives and to complete the module activities. The voice scripts were included in print, and both the PowerPoint® slides and the scripts were available to students, thus allowing for a wider variety of learning styles using voice and text. Students are divided into small groups to complete module activities. Students post ideas to a discussion board, which contains a question relating each module to the real world. An example of a small group activity is as follows: Students are given census data about a geographic community. They also view a video tour of the same community. Students are asked to develop a consensus "composite picture" of the community using both types of data. Each group can post its "composite picture" on the discussion board. Dr. G. provides synchronous office hours for one hour a week.

Another consideration is grading. Will participation be graded? If so, how does the student need to participate to earn a grade? Traditionally, Schools of Nursing are bound by approval of the curriculum committee. Do traditional and online classes have the same syllabus? Must grading be the same with both modalities? If so, how will participation be included in the online learning environment? Is grading of participation necessary to engage students in active communication during the course? Participation can be a mandatory and expected behavior in online courses. Examples of criteria for expected participation and grading can be found in the Course Management Methods chapter (Chapter 8) of this book.

Reconceptualizing Laboratory Courses

Because many nursing courses have associated laboratory experiences, consideration must be made for learning psychomotor skills. The components of the learning process for psychomotor skills that differ in traditional vs. online learning environments are practice and feedback. Traditional learners learn the procedure then attend laboratory sessions to perform the skill under the supervision of an expert, who in turn will give the students feedback on their performance. Once they master the skill in the laboratory, the student will perform the skill with a proctor and her proficiency will be evaluated. Another name for this clinical activity is called a "cognitive apprenticeship," which is discussed in further detail in the chapter on interaction (Chapter 7). Students learning in online environments can obtain the didactic material online. The challenge is to provide students with practice opportunities, feedback, and evaluation. Some options are:

- Students attend the laboratory sessions with traditional students.
- Instructors assign preceptors in the community for the students, and the preceptor gives feedback to the student.
- Students choose preceptors, and the instructor coordinates and monitors the experience while the preceptor gives feedback.
- Clinical instructors can be assigned to a geographic cohort of students; the laboratory experience is contracted with local institutions and the instructor gives feedback to the students.
- Partner with schools of nursing and contract for use of their laboratory facilities and obtain feedback from instructors.
- Contract with schools near the student that have interactive video options and laboratory facilities; students can practice using procedure guidelines using videoconferencing with the faculty member, who can give feedback via television.
- Use laptops with videoconferencing to practice skills with the instructor at a remote location, who then gives feedback.

Some options for assessing students are:

- Students can take a proficiency test administrated by the instructor at the school of nursing.
- The proficiency test can be given and assessed by their preceptor.
- The proficiency test can be administered by a preceptor, videotaped, and then assessed by the instructor.
- The student can take the proficiency test at an outreach site where an instructor will administer and assess students in a geographic cohort.

- Community resources can administer the proficiency test at an outreach site, and the instructor can assess student proficiency via live video.
- Students can use a laptop computer and videoconferencing to perform the proficiency test, with the instructor assessing from a remote site.

Reconceptualizing Clinical Courses

Some courses that are offered online have a clinical component. Clinical experiences should provide the students with guidance, mentoring, role modeling, feedback, and assessment of clinical competencies associated with the course. The following questions should be asked:

- How will guidance and mentoring be given to the student and by whom?
- Who will provide role modeling and how?
- How will the student receive feedback?
- How will the mastery of course competencies be assessed for each student?

Clinical experiences in online nursing programs can be on-site or individually arranged with preceptors. Duke University, for example, (nursing.duke.edu/modules/son_academic/index.php?id=6) requests that students complete their clinical experiences with the Duke Health System. Out-of-state and other North Carolina sites can be arranged, but these placements depend on preceptor availability, licensure, and clinical site contracts. At the Medical University of South Carolina School of Nursing (www.musc.edu/nursing/academics/masters/ne.htm), clinical experiences are individually arranged, although overnight stays may be required.

Some suggestions for providing clinical students with guidance, mentoring, and role modeling are:

- Distance-learning students enroll in the same clinical experiences as the traditional students. If students are location bound, other clinical options must be developed.

- Students have a faculty-appointed or student-selected preceptor who acts as a role model and who provides the student with experiences to accomplish the clinical objectives.
- Clustered experiences—the instructor arranges for geographically clustered, intensive experiences, (e.g., 4-day, 32- to 40-hour experiences for a cohort of students in a specific geographic location).

Videoconferencing with the instructor provides student-to-student and student-to-instructor interactions. The student can answer questions, and the faculty can observe student performance or student-patient interactions and give feedback. Logs written by students in location-bound settings and shared with the preceptor and instructor provide information for the instructor to assess student perception and progress toward meeting clinical objectives.

In summary, reconceptualizing the learning environment begins with the decision to transfer traditional course material into an online learning environment. The process of answering questions about a course and using the answers to guide the development of the online learning and communication environments will helps capitalize on the benefits of the Web and computer technology. Many opportunities exist to enhance an online course through the appropriate application of technology, such as multimedia, links, and synchronous and asynchronous discussions. Laboratory and clinical courses are challenges for designing nursing courses in an online format, but as the technology advances, current methods of offering these courses can only be improved.

REFERENCES

American Association of Colleges of Nursing. (1999). White Paper: Distance technology in nursing education. Retrieved February 3, 2008, from http://www.aacn.nche.edu/Publications/WhitePapers/whitepaper.htm

6 Designing the Online Learning Environment

CAROL A. O'NEIL

Instructional design refers to a systematic and reflective process that translates the principles of learning and instruction (the pedagogy) into plans for instructional materials, activities, information resources, and evaluation (Smith & Ragan, 2004). Instructional design answers the questions: Where are we going? How will we get there? How will we know when we get there? Smith and Ragan (2004) identified three components in the instructional design process as:

- instructional analysis (Where are we going?);
- instructional strategy (How will we get there?);
- evaluation (How will we know when we get there?).

Instructional analysis includes assessing the learner and developing learning goals and objectives. Instructional strategy includes developing, delivering, and maintaining the methods and strategies for learning. Evaluation includes using strategies to assess the student's progress toward attaining the objectives (Smith & Ragan, 2004). The design should be specific enough that it is easy to implement, but flexible enough to allow faculty to be creative.

Instructional-design theory provides guidance in developing learning environments. Instructional design is the preparation and production of learning material and includes developing objectives and goals and formulating teaching and assessment strategies. Educational theory guides design structure.

GUIDED CONSTRUCTIVISM

Guided constructivism is a combination of elements from behaviorist and constructivist theories. Behaviorism is reflected in the use of objectives that are behaviorally stated, measurable, and timed. Constructivism employs active learning strategies to engage students in the learning process through interaction and meaningful learning. How does using constructivist theory impact design? Dick and Carey (2004) created a traditional instructional design model comprising steps that are widely accepted within the cognitive learning theory community. No one constructivist theory is widely accepted. Jonassen (1999) developed one such model, but others have developed unique models as well. No universally accepted model exists that shows the process of developing a constructivist course the way Dick and Carey's does for a cognitive theory course (Brandon, 2004).

Constructivist Design

The purpose of the constructivist learning environment is to provide learning opportunities in which students construct new knowledge based on existing knowledge and experience. The learning environment should be safe, supportive, and motivating so that learners can interact, solve real-world problems, work collaboratively and meaningfully, and assess their learning (Brandon, 2004). The role of the designer is to provide the learning environment so the learners can accomplish this purpose.

In this chapter, guided constructivist theory will be used to design learning environments for nursing. Constructivists view learning as student-centered and advocate that learning objectives be developed by the learner. Although this is feasible for many disciplines, it is not always feasible for nursing. Nursing relies on learning objectives that are generated by the instructor. Objectives must be included in the design of nursing courses and will most likely be instructor-generated, a characteristic of behaviorist theory. Combining instructor-driven objectives with the constructivist view results in what is called "guided constructivism." Using the constructivist approach, the target population, the purpose, delivery designs, navigation, page layout, and interaction will be discussed. The design considerations based on the review of the literature will include:

- The target population
- The purpose and objectives
- Course organization
  - Content
  - Designs
  - Activities
  - Developing multimedia
- Navigation
- Page layout
- Interaction
  - Synchronous
  - Asynchronous
  - Discussion questions

The Target Population

The first step in course design is assessing the learners (the target population), their existing knowledge of the course material, their experience in learning in online environments, and their level of computer competence. For example, an undergraduate nursing course introducing new students to the concepts of health would be structured differently than a senior-level course in community health nursing with a clinical component. The new students may be RNs returning to school for the first time in many years. This may be the first online course some learners have taken, so they have no experience with learning online. Their technical literacy levels may be low, and they probably do not know other students in the course or program. On the other hand, the senior-level students may already have had a required technology course. They may have either taken or heard about online courses from other students, so they have a support group. They may be assigned to a clinical group with a clinical instructor who can answer questions and clarify the content that is learned online. The design for the new student would be more structured with explicit due dates for activities.

To increase socialization among new students, small groups might be included so students can share their ideas with five or six other students instead of the larger class. Because participation is so important to the learning process, including a grade for participation in the new student class is a consideration. The discussion questions would be structured differently in each class. The new students may or may not be nurses, so discussion questions might incorporate life experiences that all students can relate to. The new students may be asked to devise a composite picture of a healthy community based on their readings and personal experience, whereas the seniors might be asked to develop a nursing care plan for a multiproblem family or pregnant teens in a community. The RN to BSN students tend to use nursing lingo that the traditional BSN (non-RN) student may not understand. In a chat room discussion about using the Health Belief Model to develop a colon cancer prevention program, the RNs may be discussing colonoscopies while the non-RNs are asking, "What's that?" If the new student class comprises all RN to BSN students, the activities can be devised to incorporate nursing experience. Ask yourself who the learners are, what their experiences with online learning are, and what they know about the learning material.

Assessing learning style is also important for the designer and the learner. The instructor or course designer can provide a variety of learning activities that address the different modes of learning. The VARK, Learning Style Inventory, Multiple Intelligences, and Myers-Brigg Type Indicator outlined in the Pedagogy chapter (Chapter 2) provide the resources for assessment.

Consideration should be given to how the learner moves through the learning experience. Learning can be self-paced, where the learner independently progresses through the learning experiences.

Learners can be admitted to a series of courses or learning experiences at the same time (as a cohort). The cohort takes courses on the same schedule and ends the courses at the same time. Consider which will be most effective for your learners.

The Purpose

The objectives should be stated in measurable terms and should be succinct in communicating what the student will accomplish by the end of the learning experience. Objectives should be learner and content appropriate. Objectives for the course may be outlined in the course syllabus. These broad objectives should be broken down into manageable objectives for the learning content. For example, a course objective may be that the learner will plan, implement, and evaluate a smoking cessation program in a community group. In the module, the objective is broken down into smaller objectives, for example "the learner will describe the process of developing an implementation plan" or "the learner will define formative evaluation."

In 1995 the Innovations in Distance Education (IDE) project funded by the AT&T Foundation was launched at Pennsylvania State University. In this project, faculty worked in teams to examine issues related to the design and development of distance education programs. The outcome was "An Emerging Set of Guiding Principles and Practices for the Design and Development of Distance Education." The guiding principles for learning goals and content presentation are outlined here (Ragan, 1999):

1. Learning goals are part of the instructional design plan.
2. Specific instructional strategies and activities should be directed toward providing learners with the necessary skills, knowledge, and experience to meet the goals and objectives of the course.
3. Assessment of performance should be directed toward measuring the learning goals.
4. Faculty should be provided with the instructional design and development support they need to create and prepare instructional materials for delivery via distance education.

COURSE ORGANIZATION

The course organization is dependent on the content and the learners and answers the question: What is the best way to present the content for our learners to learn? There is no right or wrong method, but what is important is having a rationale for making decisions. The design should be easy to navigate, logical, and structured, so that content builds on previous content delivered in the course.

Content

Content is the information the learner needs to know to success-fully achieve the objectives. Considering that learners have many different learning styles, the content should be presented using many different strategies. You may question, "Why?" The answer is, "Because we can!" We can easily present content using different formats. Some examples of instructional formats to present content are: audio files, newspaper or journal articles, movie clips, video, guest speakers, interactive software, links, interviews, or text-based materials.

Content should be broken down into "chunks" and organized. The basic steps in organizing your information are to divide it into logical units, establish a hierarchy of importance and generality, use the hierarchy to structure relationships among chunks, and then analyze the functional and aesthetic success of your system (Web Style Guide, 2005). Chunks should be logical and should organize the content. Two examples of chunks are modules and units.

The chunks of information are organized into a flexible and logical format, and then they are organized into mental models. Mental models show the learner what they are learning, where they are in the course, and the relationship of each chunk in the course to other chunks. For example, an undergraduate course in gerontological nursing maybe divided into chunks called modules:

Module 1 Introduction to the aging process

Module 2 Theories of aging

Module 3 Physical, psychological, sociological, and spiritual aspects of aging

Module 4 Common health problems

Module 5 Assessing the client

Module 6 Assessing the family

Module 7 Interventions: needs and resources

Module 8 Legal issues related to aging

Module 9 Ethical issues related to aging

These chunks should be organized into mental models. One idea is to combine Modules 1 to 3 into a section that could be called "The aging process." Modules 4 to 7 could be called "Caring for the aging client and family." The final section could be "Considerations in nursing care" (Modules 8 and 9). The mental models could be the aging process, caring for aging clients, and considerations in nursing care. When the learner is navigating to module 1, the learner must pass through "the aging process," thus illustrating where the learner is in the course and what is next in the course. The repetition of the mental models will instill in the student that in gerontological nursing, the nurse assesses and implements nursing care with the client and family; finally, characteristics of the aging process and legal and ethical issues should be considered in nursing care.

Design

Once the content is conceptualized, the next step is to decide how to structure the course. Course material is usually linked from the home page so it is easy to navigate. Discrete chunks of information are organized from the home page by using banners across the top and bottom and a menu bar down the left side. Every chunk should be relevant and meaningful to the learner. The most common left side menu chunks are: course information, assignments, learning content, and discussion area. The design should provide a predetermined structure that will guide the learner through the learning environment. This design adds a structure that will help novice users navigate the materials, and seasoned users will know where to look for information. A disadvantage is that navigating is limited to forward and backward with the home page as the organizing point.

Activities

Activities support learner progression through the content material. Activities should include real world experiences and active learning strategies. Some activities are: case studies, group or individual projects, peer interaction through discussion, and active learning strategies such as collaborative problem solving or Web quests.

Multimedia

Resources and experience help determine the use of multimedia presentations. Most instructors stay with what they know and what they have, because, in general, instructors do not have the time or technical skill to develop their own multimedia presentations. Little or no information is in the literature to give guidance as to whether a multimedia presentation is more effective than a text-based presentation of content. However, it does offer an alternative way of learning for those students who prefer audio presentations.

These are the guiding principles suggested by IDE (Ragan, 1999) for instructional media and tools:

1. Instructional media and tools should support the predetermined learning goals and objectives of the learning program.
2. The technology that is used should be appropriate for the widest range of students within that program's target audience.
3. Technology should clearly enhance learning.
4. The technology used should be adequately prepared and supported in order to maximize the capabilities of instructional media and tools.

5. The design used should reflect the diversity of potential learners.
6. A systematic design model should be used to guide the selection and application of media and tools.
7. Contingency strategies for technology-related interruptions must be in place.

The general rule of thumb is that "less is more." In other words, instructors can sometimes overuse technological enhancements, which end up not enhancing the course or content at all. If overused or used incorrectly, multimedia presentations can be distracting. Animation, for example, can be effectively used to demonstrate the flow of blood through the chambers of the heart, but it can also be used inappropriately, causing your course to resemble a Las Vegas billboard.

Navigation

Using the three-click rule will help with organizing the flow of information. Get the learner where you want them to go in three clicks of the mouse. Navigation directions can be in the form of a graphic, a picture, or text. Regardless of which one is used, be consistent and place the same thing in the same location on every page. Whether it is text along the left side of the page, or text boxes strung across the bottom of the page, or icons in the center of the page and text at the bottom, continue this pattern on every page. The home link is most important in navigation, because it gets the learner back to a central place. Some "do not's" are:

■ Do not overuse bolding. It causes confusion.
■ Do not use the color blue to emphasize text because blue is associated with hypertext.
■ Do not use more than three different fonts, because it may confuse the learner.

Penn State offers a Web site (http://tlt.its.psu.edu/suggestions/research/storyboard.shtml) that offers tips on choosing fonts, storyboarding and navigating, and writing for the Web.

Page Layout

The layout of each page should be consistent, appropriate in look and feel, and have a user-friendly interface (Learning to Learn, n.d.). Consistency means using the same layout on each page; that includes color, background, fonts, headings, text layout, and navigation cues. The graphic design should be fun, professional, simple, high-tech, and slick. The design is a reflection of the organization and should be professional, but it should also be functional and easy to use. Too much information on a page can make the page look cluttered and can interfere with what the learner should learn. Ask yourself how each piece of information on a page will help the learner learn.

The basic page layout includes links that are color coded and positioned in the same place on every page. Each page should have a title at the top that describes what is on the page. Here are some additional tips on page layout:

- Use headings, bolding, bullets, and graphics to emphasize important information and use them consistently.
- Group information into logical units or chunks and be consistent in the groupings.
- Look at each page through the eyes of the learner and visualize the flow of information.

The home page should include information that the learner needs to begin the learning process. The vital data that should be on the home page are: a link to course information; instructor name, contact information and a picture; a welcome message from the instructor either in text or streaming audio; and the required textbook and how to obtain it (ALN, 2000).

Interacting

Synchronous interaction requires participation with others at the same time, such as chat rooms and audio or videoconferencing. Asynchronous interactions such as bulletin boards or electronic mail lists are not time-dependent.

Students should have four types of asynchronous interactions (Learning to Learn, n.d.). There should be a forum in which learners can introduce themselves. The forum can be based on a general question such as "What would you like to tell us about yourself," or more specific, such as "When did you realize that you wanted to be a nurse?" for first-year nursing students. The introductory forum provides an opportunity for learners to find out what they have in common. If it is possible, learners should provide a picture of themselves. The instructor should always provide a picture. These activities enhance bonding and start building learning communities. The second forum is to obtain help, and a forum labeled "Technical Questions" should be provided. Student comments in this forum should be read and referred to appropriate resources or technical support team. The third type of forum is a content forum, which is used to discuss experiences with the course material. The fourth is a student lounge or a "virtual cafe" which is used for discussions not related to the course.

Discussion questions should be used to stimulate interaction among students and instructors. These questions should be open-ended and based on the relevant course content. These questions should stimulate student thinking and facilitate students learning from each other. For example, "How would you apply the principles from Unit 1 to your area of interest in nursing?" When done correctly, the answers to discussion questions will end in yet another question, thereby bringing the discussion to a higher level. For example, the student may end by saying, "Have others had a different experience?" Often it is necessary for the instructor to model this type of answer by offering their own experiences for the students to follow.

These guiding principles suggested by IDE (Ragan, 1999) for interaction are helpful:

1. Interaction among learners should be frequent and meaningful and should occur between learners and instructional materials, and between learners and the instructor.
2. Participants should build confidence and competence with the learning process and supporting technologies.
3. Create and maintain learning communities for learners.

4. Use creative solutions to complete the objectives, to maintain interaction among faculty, students, and peers and to provide access to advising and academic support services and resources.
5. Encourage and support social interactions between and among learners.

"A Course Design Model," developed by Margaret Chambers, Director of the Institute of Distance Education at the University of Maryland University College and the Web Initiative in Teaching Project instituted by the University System of Maryland from 1998 to 2002, outlines the following phases and components:

Phase One

Mapping: identify goals, issues and constraints

Architecture: reconceptualize the course and restructure into modules or educational objects

Prototype: design a sample-learning module illustrating the design decisions

Phase Two

Early Development: develop key elements, modules, or educational objects for testing with students

Field Testing: try out critical elements with real students and colleagues

Late Development: complete courseware

Phase Three:

Institutional launch: arrange for course listing, marketing and registration: post a course review site

Pilot Course Delivery: teach the course online with external peer reviewers

Revision: modify and update.

DEVELOPING AN ONLINE COURSE

To facilitate the course design process, ALN (2000) suggests "The Yellow Sticky Method." The steps in that process are as follows:

1. Gather pads of yellow stickies (Post-It Notes®), a large piece of paper (or whiteboard), and a pen or marker.
2. On a sticky write "Homepage" and place it on the large piece of paper or whiteboard.
3. Consider your course platform, such as Angel or Blackboard, and write the key elements of your platform, each on a separate sticky. For example: syllabus, content (mental models), course material, communication, and assignments—and then organize them into a logical format on the large piece of paper or whiteboard.
4. Think how the course should be organized. Move stickies around until you create the structure that makes most sense to you.
5. Use the pen or marker and draw lines to connect the pages and sections.
6. Focus on the "microlevel"—specific lectures and readings; create a sticky for each lecture, assignment, and quiz, and organize them on the board.
7. Consider learning strategies that you will use to disseminate the content.

ALN (2000) suggests a quality check: Examine the pages you have created to check that the major features are in place, that a clear and consistent navigational structure exists, and that the assignments, assessment criteria, and learning strategies are in place and adequate for students to reach the course goals.

IDE (Ragan, 1999) also offers guiding principles for assessment, measurement, and learner services and support, to be considered in designing online learning environments. These are the assessment and measurement principles:

1. Assessment instruments and activities should be congruent with the learner's learning goals and skills.

2. Assessment and measurement strategies should enable the learner to assess their progress through the learning experience.

3. Assessment and measurement strategies should accommodate the special needs, characteristics, and situations of the learner.

4. Learners should have ample opportunities and accessible methods for providing feedback.

These are the guiding principles for learner services and support:

1. A comprehensive system of technical support services should be in place to ensure the effective use of technologies in distance education programming for learners, instructors, and staff.

2. Faculty should have access to adequate support in instructional technology and distance-education methodologies.

3. Support systems should be designed to provide service seven days a week, twenty-four hours a day for faculty and learners.

4. Regular feedback mechanisms should be designed and implemented to assess the successes and failures of the various support services.

In summary, design begins with an assessment of the learner and the technological expertise of the developer. Begin design with behavioral objectives that are appropriate to the learner and based on the content. The structure is dependent on the software platform, but regardless of the "givens," multiple methods of learning should be included to accommodate various student learning styles. The learner can navigate via graphics or text, but should be able to get where she wants to go in three clicks (or less) of the mouse. The layout of every page should be identical and follow a template so the learner knows where she is on a page and how to navigate to somewhere else. Learners need to communicate with each other and with the instructor. The most common form of communication is through bulletin boards, but there are other means of interacting, such as through chat rooms and audio and videoconferencing.

REFERENCES

Asynchronous Learning Networks (ALN) (2000). Pre-conference workshop: Strategic planning for on-line courses. ALN Conference at University of Maryland, University College, July, 2000.

Adaptive Technology Resource Centre (ATRC) (2008). Learning to learn: About Web-based instructional design. Retrieved January 22, 2008, from http://snow.utoronto.ca/Learn2/design.html

Brandon, Bill (2004). Applying instructional systems processes to constructivist learning environments. *The e-Learning Developers' Journal,* June 29. Retrieved February 8, 2008, from http://www.elearningguild.com/pdf/2/062904DES.pdf

Dick, W., Carey, L., Carey, J. (2004). Systematic design of instruction. New York: Addison-Wesley, Longman.

Jonassen, D. (1999). Designing constructivist learning environments. In Reigeluth, C. (ed.). *Instructional-design theories and models: A new paradigm of instructional theory.* Volume II. Mahwah, NJ: Lawrence Erlbaum Associates.

Ragan, L. (1999). Good teaching is good teaching: An emerging set of guiding principles and practices for the design and development of education. *Cause/Effect,* 22(1), 20–24.

Smith, P. L. & Ragan, T. J. (2004). *Instructional design.* New York: John Wiley & Sons.

Web Style Guide. (2005). Retrieved February 4, 2008, from http://www.webstyleguide.com/site/organize.html

7

Interacting and Communicating Online

CHERYL A. FISHER

Instructional interactivity takes place among the instructor, the learners, and the content (Figure 7.1), and each interaction must be considered in the instructional design. In a traditional classroom, communication between the teacher and student and between students is generally synchronous (occurring at the same time and place). In distance learning, communication can be synchronous or asynchronous (not occurring at the same time). This chapter will discuss different types of interaction and communication that are well-suited for distance courses.

IMPORTANCE OF INTERACTION

A successful online course is easy to access, easy to navigate, and makes it easy to interact with others. Interactivity means more than just clicking a mouse button to advance to the next page. Interactivity requires meaningful feedback (i.e., leading toward an established goal) for each learner. Often this involves written confirmation of a correct response, or a dialog with the instructor or other learners. In

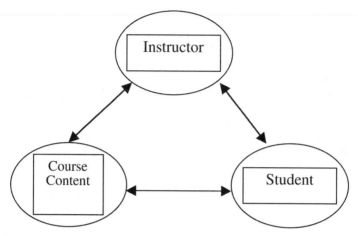

Figure 7.1 Elements of interaction in online learning environments.

the online environment, interaction can take place in the form of a question and answer session, an essay, or a discussion, and may be asynchronous or synchronous.

Characteristics of a "good" online conversation, according to Sherry, Traralin, and Billig (2000), include evidence of problem solving, informed decision making, and depth of both student-and teacher-facilitated discussions. There should also be evidence of episodes that extend the conversation beyond a simple question-and-answer interaction to the examination of complex problems from multiple perspectives. For example, if a discussion were started on the topic of bioterrorism, the facilitator should try to elicit comments from an acute care and a community health nursing perspective. The questions should be open-ended and require students to hypothesize and develop their own questions on the subject.

Wilson (2003) suggests that the electronic environment can be structured for online interaction as a flexible model of learning. The online environment can be structured for effective social constructivist learning utilizing interactive online discussion. These models of collaborative learning are becoming mandatory in course design and delivery as online learning is incorporated into institutional policies.

Giguere, Formica and Harding (2004), who studied interaction and professional development, found that interaction had less to do with personal interaction (e.g., building a community of learners) and more to do with providing a means of reinforcing various elements from the content of the training. Research studies have suggested that learning in groups improves students' achievement of learning objectives. Little investigation, however, has been done to compare the effects of different types of interaction (peer-to-peer, student-to-instructor) on learning in distance learning environments.

ASYNCHRONOUS COMMUNICATION

Asynchronous communication occurs at different times. It is characterized by time-independence, meaning the sender and receiver communicate with time delays. When preparing online courses, instructors build into the instructional design mechanisms asynchronous instructor-to-student interaction and communication.

Asynchronous communication uses the Internet for e-mail, electronic bulletin boards, or Web-based software. E-mail allows for personal, private communication. The electronic bulletin board is used for all participants to post and read messages. This form of asynchronous communication is most commonly used in main discussion areas of online classrooms and allows students to interact with faculty, other students, and course content.

Instructor-to-Student Interactions

Picciano (2001) suggests that instructor and student interaction with course content compose critical elements of learning. In traditional environments, textbooks, notes written on chalkboards, diagrams shown on overhead projectors, slide shows, and video clips compose the instructional content for a class (Picciano, 2001). In distance courses, instructors can decide how best to deliver course content along with the guidance of an instructional designer. More sophisticated delivery modes are becoming popular as increased bandwidth allows for the downloading of multimedia files, Power Point® or Flash® presentations (with or without associated audio), and streaming video. However, the instructor should not convert materials used in traditional courses without considering how distance technologies can allow the course materials to be used more effectively and efficiently. Additionally, the instructor needs to consider whether the students are able to access multimedia requiring plug-ins for viewing and to access large data files. Since many students still access the Internet using dial-up modems, the time required to download large files should be supplemented with a smaller file option (i.e., a text version of an audio file). Doing this will allow the students to have options for accessing course information based on preference and bandwidth capability.

Depending on how the technology is used, students may find it easier to use or interact with distance learning content than traditional classroom content. Instructor notes or slides available for print from the course site allow students to take notes more thoroughly while listening to online lectures.

Graphics or animated images available online can be viewed over and over by students without having to go to the library or nursing lab. Animated graphics create simulations to demonstrate blood flow or actions of the cranial nerves and help students visualize body processes better than a one-dimensional textbook is capable of showing.

Student-to-Student Interactions

Student-to-student interaction using asynchronous communication can take place in the main discussion area of an online course or in collaborative groups. The main discussion area of an online course should be analogous to the main classroom in a face-to-face course. This discussion area is where the students and instructor should meet to participate in active dialogue and discuss course material. It is also where students have the opportunity to learn from each other and ask questions for further understanding of course content. Picciano (2001) suggests that it is this interaction that is an important component of the learning dynamic. Technology is responsible for bringing students together, and because it takes some extra effort, the result is actually more interaction (Gilbert, 2001). Since students cannot hide in an online course, especially when drawn into interaction by the instructor, the result is active participation that is often not observed in a face-to-face classroom. Students often feel less inhibited and have time to collect their thoughts prior to speaking up in an asynchronous discussion.

Group Collaboration

Groups or learning teams are another means by which the instructor can promote collaboration and interaction in the online classroom. Creating teams is useful for the purpose of small group discussion, completion of group assignments, engagement in small group activities, and simulations (Palloff & Pratt, 1999). Teams can be formed by offering students the opportunity to self-select membership or by instructor assignment. Sometimes students like to work together based on past experience and sometimes by time zones. Once groups are formed, it is important to post guidelines and expectations of team performance. For example:

1. Each team will designate, elect, or appoint a team coordinator or leader.
2. The leader will remain the same throughout the course unless replaced by a majority vote of the team or by the instructor.
3. The team leader may make a decision unless overruled by a majority.
4. Any project assigned to the group will receive a grade that applies to every member of that group.
5. The team leader will have the final authority to modify any team member's grade up or down (except for her own).
6. The instructor will have the final say in all cases where the team cannot reach a decision.

Within these guidelines it is expected that the team members will evaluate each other's work, participate, and contribute to the team assignment. Team self-evaluation is an option to offer teams to help promote a productive work environment.

SYNCHRONOUS COMMUNICATION

Synchronous communication can take place in the form of live chat rooms or interactive videoconferencing. The greatest challenge faced with synchronous communication or meetings is to coordinate a time when all participants are available. Considerations that need to be made are differences in time zones and students working different shifts. Students often request that a live chat section of the course be available because it reduces feelings of isolation. However, it is rarely a productive discussion and frequently disintegrates into simple one-line contributions of minimal depth. Palloff and Pratt (1999) describe how chat sessions can replicate face-to-face classroom discussion, but in fact it is probably the fastest typist who will contribute the greatest amount to the discussion. Additionally, synchronous discussion can rapidly get out of sync because if a slower typist responds to a comment after several other points have been made, the responses no longer follow in order. Guidelines for participation should be established from the start so that the students have clear expectations of how the chat room will work. Some instructors prefer to use the synchronous chat feature of the classroom for office hours only. This gives the student the opportunity to interact with the instructor in real time and have any pertinent questions answered immediately.

The logistics of timing a live chat meeting can truly be reason enough not to use them. If students are working shifts in different time zones, it may be impossible to find a time that is convenient for all. Nurses working the night shift may have to get up in the middle of the day to participate. This will lead to reduced quality in their contributions and disruption in sleep prior to going back to work. When students are dispersed internationally, the window for meeting times is again reduced.

In the online environment, net meetings using Web cameras can be used, but this technology currently works best for small numbers of individuals. Synchronous video conferencing requires students to be at a certain place at a certain time and is not yet advanced enough to be used in online courses. Possibilities for actual participation in lectures offered in remote places exist, but may require that the student visit a campus that has the video conferencing technology in place. This technology allows students in several locations to share the same learning experience simultaneously through two-way video and audio.

BUILDING COMMUNITY

Regardless of whether you use asynchronous or synchronous communication in the online classroom, the students should feel as if they are a part of the learning community. Distance students often feel isolated and alone in their early experiences online, but with proper guidance and personalized attention, they quickly bond and come to depend on each other for learning and moral support. It is the instructor's responsibility for facilitating the personal and social aspects of an online community in order to create a successful learning experience (Palloff & Pratt, 1999). Collins and Berge (1996) write that promoting human relationships by affirming and recognizing students' input, providing opportunities for students to develop a sense of group cohesiveness, maintaining the group as a unit, and helping members to work together for a mutual goal are necessary elements for building community in an online environment.

So how does an instructor begin to develop a sense of community in an online course? Many begin with introductions or an initial request for posting of a biography. The instructor can model how the "bio" is to be posted by posting one first and asking for (1) professional experiences, (2) educational background, and (3) personal information. The bios will allow students to find commonalities and provide students the opportunity to get to know each other. Another technique may be to use ice breakers. Online ice breakers can include games or strategies to get students to talk about themselves; for example, "the ABC's of me" or "post eight nouns about yourself." These ice breakers allow students to seek others in the class with similar interests or experiences that may facilitate good working relationships. Another strategy for facilitating community is to set up an area called cyber-chat or a student lounge where students can meet and greet without loading up the main classroom with personal chatter.

New generations of social software show a human face online and help students and faculty communicate, educate, and interact with their communities. These new software tools include blogs, wikis, social networking software, photo sharing, podcasting, and more. The ease of use and popularity of these new communication methodologies have potential for tremendous impact (Farkas, 2007).

Active Learning

In order to actively engage learners in the online learning process and to facilitate the meaning-making process that is a part of the constructivist approach through which this learning occurs, the content of the course should be embedded in everyday life (Palloff & Pratt, 1999). In other words, the more learners can relate their life experience and what they already know to the context of the online classroom, the deeper their understanding will be of what they learn. In nursing, for example, students should be provided case-based scenarios or problems to resolve based on their area of interest in nursing.

The online instructor can promote active learning through the creative use of instructional design strategies. For example, the incorporation of Web quests or problem-based learning scenarios will facilitate meaningful active learning and help students search for real life answers. A Web quest is an inquiry-oriented activity in which some or all of the information that learners interact with comes from resources on the Internet (Dodge, 1997). Web quests can be of either short or long duration and are deliberately designed to make the best use of a learner's time. Web quests should contain at least the following parts:

- An introduction that sets the stage and provides some background information.
- A task that is doable and interesting.
- A set of information sources needed to complete the task. Many (though not necessarily all) of the resources are embedded in

the Web quest document itself as anchors pointing to information on the World Wide Web. Information sources might include Web documents, experts available via e-mail or real-time conferencing, searchable databases on the net, and books and other documents physically available in the learner's setting. Because pointers to resources are included, the learner is not left to wander through Web space completely adrift.

- A description of the process the learners should go through in accomplishing the task. The process should be broken down into clearly described steps.
- Some guidance on how to organize the information acquired. This may take the form of guiding questions or directions to complete organizational frameworks such as timelines, concept maps, or cause-and-effect diagrams.
- A conclusion that brings closure to the quest, reminds the learners about what they've learned, and perhaps encourages them to extend the experience into other domains.

Several examples of nursing Web quests are available on the web. An example is one WebQuest that provides nursing students with a challenge related to Type 2 Diabetes: "Community Health Nurses, Older Southern Women & Their Good Cookin." This WebQuest combined several challenges for the students by incorporating a disease process (diabetes), persons affected by the disease process (a group of older women living in the south), and a challenge (a culture built around a style of cooking that is incompatible with management of diabetes).

Problem-based learning (PBL) using case-based scenarios are another example of active learning strategies that can be used by instructors to promote collaboration among teams of students. PBL is an instructional method that challenges students to "learn to learn," working cooperatively in groups to seek solutions to real world problems. These problems are used to engage students' curiosity and initiate learning the subject matter. PBL prepares students to think critically and analytically, and to find and use appropriate learning resources. With its roots in the medical profession, PBL was originally developed to assist interns to determine a diagnosis based on the given symptoms of a patient. An example of a PBL scenario is "Whose Embryo Is It, Anyway?," found on the University of Delaware Web site (www.udel.edu/inst/problems/embryo). This case involves an ethical decision based on a mix-up at a fertility clinic. This example presents a case based on a real example and follows with four group discussion questions that require research and inquiry to answer.

Design characteristics of PBL include:

1. Reliance on problems to drive the curriculum—the problems do not test skills; they assist in development of the skills themselves.
2. The problems are truly ill-structured—there is not meant to be one solution, and as new information is gathered in a reiterative process, perception of the problem changes, and thus the solution changes.
3. Students solve the problems—teachers are coaches and facilitators.
4. Students are only given guidelines for how to approach problems—there is no single formula for student approaches to the problem.
5. Authentic, performance-based assessment—there is a seamless start and end of the instruction. (Savery & Duffy 1991).

Once students are confronted with a real world scenario, they should be prompted to ask:

- What do I already know about this problem or question?
- What do I need to know to effectively address this problem or question?
- What resources can I access to determine a proposed solution or hypothesis?

When the students have clearly defined the problem, they may choose to access human or electronic information resources. They may also need to evaluate the resources by asking how current the information is, how credible and accurate it is, and if there is any reason to suspect bias in the source. Because there is no assigned text in this activity, students are forced to use the Internet as the primary research tool and to critically evaluate the information they find. In the final stage, students construct a solution to the problem. Students may create a multimedia production, or a more traditional written paper focused around an essential question. This activity forces students to organize information in new ways and helps them develop new tools or strategies for solving real-world problems. In addition to developing problem-solving skills, Savery and Duffy (1991) acknowledge that students also develop skills in self-directed learning and team participation.

Cognitive apprenticeship is another strategy that involves close communication between experts and novices in an authentic context. Nurses taking clinical courses in community health, adult health, or other practical areas will need to be involved in this type of learning experience. In this environment, novices progress along a path to expertise by refining authentic products and processes under the mentorship of experts (Sherry, Traralin, & Billig, 2000). As with any apprenticeship, this involves observation of experts in action, coaching of novices by experts, and successive approximation to expert work as novices gain expertise. The students may be physically present in a hospital or community to develop skills while participating in the didactic part of the course online. Ongoing dialogue and conversations between and among students and instructors will help students to identify problems that they may encounter or skills that they need to develop.

In summary, interaction and communication has been identified as the core of the course where learning takes place in an online environment. It is the interaction between instructors, students and the course content that is necessary in order for the content to be applied and knowledge to be developed. Group activities and active learning techniques should be applied and are characteristic of a constructivist-learning environment. Web quests, problem-based learning, and cognitive apprenticeships are examples of active learning strategies that are well suited to the online classroom and will work well with online nursing courses.

REFERENCES

Collins, M. & Berge. Z. (1996). Facilitating interaction in computer mediated online courses. Retrieved April 3, 2008, from http://www.emoderators.com/moderators/flcc.html

Dodge, B. (1997). Web Quests: A technique for internet-based learning. *Distance Educator,* 1(2), 10–13.

Farkas, M. (2007). Social software in libraries: Building collaboration, communication, and community online. Medford, NJ: Information Today, Inc

Giguere, P., Formica, S., Harding, W. (2004). Large-scale interaction strategies for Web-based professional development. *American Journal of Distance Education,* 18(4), 207–223.

Gilbert, S. D. (2001). *How to be a successful online student.* New York: McGraw Hill Professional.

Moore, M. (1993). Transactional distance theory. In D. Keegan. (ed). *Theoretical Principles of Distance Education.* New York: Routledge.

Palloff, R. & Pratt, K. (1999). *Building learning communities in cyberspace: Effective strategies for the online classroom.* San-Francisco: Jossey-Bass.

Picciano, A. (2001). *Distance learning: Making connections across virtual space and time.* Old Tappen, NJ: Prentice Hall

Savery, J., & Duffy, T. (1991). Problem-based learning. In B. Wilson, *Constructivist learning environments: Case studies in instructional design* (pp. 135–146). Englewood Cliffs, NJ: Educational Technology Publications.

Sherry, L., Traralin, F., & Billig, S. (2000). Good online conversation: Building on research to inform practice. *Journal of Interactive Learning Research,* 11(1), 85–127.

Vygotsky, L. (1978). *Mind in society: The development of higher psychological processes.* Cambridge, MA: Harvard University Press.

Wilson, S. (2003). Online interaction impacts learning: Teaching the teacher to teach online. *Interact, Integrate, Impact.* Retrieved April 26, 2008, from http://www.ascilite.org.au/conferences/adelaide03/docs/backup/541.pdf

8

Course Management Methods

CHERYL A. FISHER

Many instructors around the world are discovering the exciting potential of the online environment to deliver high quality instruction to people who would otherwise not be able to participate in higher education. This presents an exciting and challenging opportunity for collaborative learning and is affecting the way traditional classes are taught. Managing an online course can have many similarities to managing a face-to-face course but may differ in complexity with the use of technology and the geographic distance.

Facilitating learning at a distance requires faculty to take some new approaches to managing the teaching and learning process. The faculty role in the online classroom requires greater attention to detail, structure, and monitoring of student activity. According to Kimball (2002), effective faculty have a completely new mind-set about technology and must learn to manage a new set of variables that determine the extent to which their courses are effective. In this chapter, the role of the instructor in planning, organizing, and managing the online learning environment, along with the expectations of the student, will be discussed.

FACULTY ROLE

The role of the instructor shifts from the traditional classroom "sage on the stage" to the "guide on the side." Although these might be overused phrases, there is a lot of truth to them as they apply to the instructor role shift that takes place when teaching online. In addition to technological and pedagogical changes, research substantiates that the evolving distance-learning phenomena has an impact on the role of faculty (Ryan, Carlton, & Ali, 2004). In a traditional setting, the instructor feeds information to students in a lecture or PowerPoint® slide presentation format. This method of teaching has long been used in educational settings and has come to be what most students expect. In a distance learning role, the instructor focuses on discussing and reviewing materials presented through video and audio technologies, assigned readings, and interactive group activities. The faculty role is that of content expert, who guides or facilitates student learning through direction to resources and stimulation of discussion.

A trained facilitator is an important component of an online program. Oftentimes, the facilitator is also the course designer and responsible for monitoring the online course. In this role, the facilitator can influence the success or failure of the course. The facilitator's training, personality, professionalism, and knowledge of the content become important factors influencing the online classroom.

According to the Illinois Online Network (ION, 2008), "This brings new pressures on instructors, both to deal with a different way of teaching and to interact with and manage a 24-hour-a-day classroom populated by adults who demand relevance and may require extra support due to their already busy lives." Some responsibilities include:

- Planning and organizing the course;
- Creating a collaborative atmosphere;
- Providing opportunities for teamwork;
- Constructing open-ended, thought-provoking questions;
- Providing direction and leadership;
- Setting the agenda;

- Giving feedback and reinforcement;
- Sequencing content and pacing the material.

In order to perform these responsibilities, successful online faculty should have some basic background knowledge and preparation to teach online. According to ION (2008), the instructor should:

- Have a broad base of life experiences in addition to academic credentials in the subject matter. This will enable the instructor to actively participate with students and guide their constructive thinking.
- Be open, concerned, flexible, and sincere so she can compensate for the lack of physical presence.
- Feel comfortable communicating in writing, because this is the basic element of the process.
- Believe that learning can occur in facilitated online learning environments.
- Believe that the online learning process includes learning information that can be used today and that requires critical thinking.
- Be supportive of the development of critical thinking. Have the appropriate credentials to teach the subject. Be well trained in teaching and learning online.

PLANNING AND ORGANIZING

When planning and organizing an online course, the instructor must look at the overall course in terms of objectives, outcomes, assessment, and evaluation. The planning should include the criteria discussed in the reconceptualization chapter of this book (Chapter 5). The instructor should keep in mind that it is in this beginning phase of course development where the expertise of an instructional designer and an information technology expert should be employed.

The curriculum of an online program must be designed especially for the collaborative nature of online learning. Course content should be organized in modules with clear deadlines for the assigned work in each section. These concise lectures should be compensated with open-ended remarks and discussion questions that will elicit comments and provide the students opportunities to contribute varying viewpoints. The curriculum should focus on applying knowledge utilizing real world examples and fostering critical thinking skills within the opportunities of exchanging ideas. Instructors should give clear and simple assignments with clear instructions.

Collaboration

Once the course has been planned and organized, the instructor is ready to launch the course. It is now the instructor's responsibility to create a collaborative atmosphere. To create this environment, the students should encounter a friendly, welcoming message as they first enter the online course. Using an "ice breaker" such as requesting a short biography as the initial assignment will give students something to which they can respond. The instructor can post his or her bio first as an introduction and then ask the students to present theirs in a similar format. For example, the instructor can describe work experiences, educational background, course expectations, and some personal information. This is not only a way of introducing oneself to the class but also a way for the instructor to gain information about students that can be used later in class discussions. The students often find that they have similar backgrounds or professional interests, which then allows them to begin developing a sense of community through realization of shared goals and shared expectations of the course. By asking the learners to contribute their goals and expectations, the instructor is able to determine if her approach to the course will correspond more closely to the needs of the learners.

Students should be encouraged to respond to each other's postings. The best way to teach students how to post meaningful statements is for the instructor to model how they should respond. Modeling a short but welcoming response does this best. Not only does this enable students to begin opening up to each other, but it begins creating a safe space in which they can interact. The posting of an introduction is the first step in revealing who one is to the others in the class, and it is critical that they feel acknowledged so they can continue to do that safely throughout the duration of the course. This is the first point of connection—the point where these important relationships begin to develop (Palloff & Pratt, 1999).

Developing Discussion Questions

Developing or creating open-ended questions is the primary method for stimulating discussion, assessing student learning, and providing for interactivity amongst the learners. The discussion questions should be based on the desired learning outcomes and can vary in number based on instructor preference. The discussion questions should be open ended, thought provoking, and relevant to student learning. Then, the instructor as well as the students must learn the art of expansive questions in order to keep the discussion going. This allows the responsibility for facilitation of discussion to be shared among all participants. And finally, students should be encouraged to provide constructive feedback to one another throughout the course. Rather than being at the forefront of the discussion, the instructor is an equal player, acting as a gentle guide (Palloff & Pratt, 1999). The sharing of this responsibility among the participants is one way instructors can stretch their facilitative skills.

The discussion questions should be developed in a way that there is not a right or wrong answer. They serve to stimulate thinking and are a means by which the instructor can assess student learning and understanding of the issues. The instructor needs to model this form of questioning so that students can learn to answer questions in a substantive manner, provide an example, cite a resource, and end with an expansive question for his classmates. This allows for the discussion to progress to a higher level as questions are answered and expanded upon by students pursuing the issue. The instructor's role is to closely monitor the discussion and to jump in with another question, thereby expanding the level of thinking beyond the original question. A poor or minimal response to a question could indicate that student thinking has not been stimulated and that the learners have not been compelled or inspired to respond. Commenting on discussion questions by asking students for more information or by sharing some aspects of their professional expertise can help to engage students and facilitate online discussions.

Direction and Leadership

Providing direction and leadership in an online course should begin before the students enter the classroom. The syllabus or a separate document on how to run the course should be used to provide clear directions for students about the following aspects of the course:

- General information
- Contact information
- Textbooks or other course materials
- Course requirements
- Where to start
- How I plan to run this course
- Class schedule, parts of the classroom
- Group work and expectations
- Technical support
- Grading
- Student responsibility

A sample syllabus is included at the end of this chapter (Exhibit 8.1). General course information should include course start and end dates, project due dates, and midterm and final exam dates.

Time off for spring break or other breaks related to holidays or official closing of the university should also be included on the course calendar. Contact information is important for students in order to have easy access to faculty. Often it is helpful to put a primary and a secondary e-mail address, work and home phone numbers (optional), and the best times to make contact. Times of contact are important, especially when students are working shifts and faculty may be located in a different time zone.

Required texts and supporting documents should be available to students before class begins or at least during the first week of class. Students should have the ability to order books from either the bookstore or another online book service such as Amazon.com. Other recommended texts should be listed in case students are interested in purchasing these as well.

Course requirements help students know in advance what they will need to do and what faculty has identified as requirements to complete this course; for example: view lecture material, assigned readings, participate in team exercises, complete assignments, and take midterm and final examinations. Listing requirements ahead of time will help students organize their approach to the course and will provide clarity of course requirements.

"Where to Start" and "How I Plan to Run This Course" are opportunities to help students begin. Often, in a face-to-face course, this is the housekeeping session that takes place on the first day of class. When directing students where to start, it is critical to have students attend either a face-to-face or an online orientation. It is in this orientation that they will be instructed to obtain a password for the course and begin to learn basic navigation of the courseware if this is their first experience with online learning. Once students are inside the online course, they should be directed to read the course information carefully. This should include the syllabus and all supporting documents that will be used to run the course.

The course schedule can be placed in a calendar and should include important dates that students should note. For example, weekly lectures and discussion questions will be posted every Monday. Discussion question answers should be posted by Wednesday; weekly or module summaries should be posted by Friday. This schedule will help students develop some structure for their learning and help them to juggle their workload. Let them know when quizzes will be posted, and again take the opportunity to highlight due dates of midterms, final exams, and papers. One lesson for faculty that cannot be overstated is that *you cannot be too redundant in the online environment*. The more places a student can find important dates, the better. The main parts of the classroom should also be clearly delineated. If using courseware such as Blackboard or WebCT, the left menu bar is a good place to start designing the online classroom.

For example:

Announcements: Frequent communications and important dates to remember should be posted here.

Course Information: This section should contain documents such as the syllabus, course packet, quizzes, sample APA-formatted paper (or whatever style guide is required), instructions on submitting assignments and more.

Faculty Information: This section should contain contact information (as above) as well as other contact information that might be useful while students are enrolled in your course.

Assignments: This section should contain instructions for individual assignments and the grading criteria.

Course Documents: This section houses course lectures, course objectives, readings, and supplemental Web links for each lecture of the course. This is the primary location for the course content.

Student Tools: This is where the digital drop box, student grades, calendar, and other tools are located.

By identifying the parts of the online classroom, orientation information is restated and a text document is provided for reference. Once this document is written, it is highly reusable except for dates or changes that have taken place in the course. Technical support contact information should also be provided in the form of hours of availability, phone numbers, and e-mail. Although this information is provided, invariably technical questions will show up in the discussion area of the classroom. Posting a message thread for technical questions will often allow students to answer each other's questions and keep the questions separate from the course content of the main classroom. This section could be titled "Cyber Café" and would provide students with a place for general course questions.

Grading information should also be clearly delineated in terms of: (1) methods of evaluation (i.e., class exercises, assignments, papers, and exams), and (2) criteria for the final grade. For example:

Participation 10%

Team Exercises 30%

Midterm Exam 30%

Final Exam 30%

Total 100%

Just as in face-to-face classes, students need to know the weight of graded assignments. They should also know what percentage or point value is required for letter grade. This is also a good place to include the policy on late assignments (regarding point reduction) or incomplete grades, and information about the university's policy on academic integrity.

One aspect of ensuring quality and academic integrity is finding ways to document student identity as related to course assignments and testing. In short, faculty need to be sure that individuals receiving course credit are, indeed, the individuals who do the work. Institutions have a variety of ways to achieve identity security in the context of a meaningful assessment. The choices that an institution has will depend on the institutional resources, the type of assessment appropriate for measuring achievement of the learning objectives, and the number of students that need to be served. While high-tech methodologies exist for secure identification, such as retinal scanning or facial, voice, or fingerprint identification, institutions may not be ready to invest in these technologies. Another alternative is proctored testing centers or Web-based testing software. This software requires a user name and password and can provide a different test each time the user logs in.

Setting the Agenda

The course agenda includes the nonnegotiable parts of the course (i.e., those things that cannot be changed). The course agenda allows the student to anticipate what to expect from the course in terms of an overall preview. On a more detailed level, an agenda should provide students with information about what to expect on a weekly basis. The overall course agenda could be incorporated into the syllabus and the course calendar and could include information such as objectives, due dates of assignments, midterms, and finals. The overall agenda will allow students to organize their time around important dates and course deliverables. The weekly agenda will allow students to organize their week. For example, at the beginning of every week the instructor could post the weekly objectives, the reading assignments, and the individual and group assignments. By having these agenda items available, the students will be unlikely to miss any important information that is necessary for course completion. Do not hesitate to repeat instructions and post assignment reminders of deadlines, as this can be very helpful for students.

Sequence and Pace

The sequence and pace of providing lectures and assignments can be left to the instructor's discretion. Some instructors prefer to post lectures, assignments, and discussion questions on a week-by-week basis. This controls the pace of the course and does not allow the students to work ahead. This model would most closely replicate the sequence and pace of a face-to-face classroom. Some instructors like to guide the online classroom discussion using this strategy. Another option would be to release course content by units, clusters, or modules. Using this strategy, the instructor would still want to control the discussion by posting discussion questions regularly within the block of time designated for a particular unit. A third strategy for sequencing the release of course content would be to give the student the entire course at the beginning of class. Students will be required to participate according to the instructor's instructions. This strategy allows students to work ahead in their reading, writing, and group work, but also allows the instructor to control the collaborative learning in the main discussion area of the classroom. Some instructors have found it useful to put start and stop dates on discussions. For example, if a particular discussion thread is only going to be open for two weeks, the instructor should post start and stop dates at the beginning of the message thread so that students know when to move on to the next topic.

Feedback

Feedback is one of the most critical activities that instructors need to be aware of in online learning because of the lack of face-to-face interaction. Feedback goes beyond confirmation of correct answers.

Feedback is necessary for students to develop new understandings and to facilitate learning (Perrin, 1999). Students need much more support and feedback in the online environment than in a traditional course (ION, 2008). It is necessary for instructors to respond to students in a timely manner (usually within 24–48 hours) in order for students to feel encouraged to participate and to continue to participate at a high level. Online students need extra reinforcement and verification of their performance. Positive feedback, constructive feedback, and tone are all areas that instructors need to be aware of and sensitive to when responding to students. For example, proposing an alternative viewpoint might be interpreted by a student as an incorrect statement on his part as opposed to just an expansion of ideas. While maintaining a positive and encouraging tone and keeping things light with humor and emoticons, the instructor can still maintain a professional atmosphere in the class environment.

Most instructors know that communicating with students can positively influence learning and can be done using feedback techniques. Because improvement in learning is more likely to occur following both written and oral critiques of student work, it is important to provide more than just a number or letter grade on student assignments. Written critiques or telephone conversations can be provided to students for more in-depth explanations of grades, but more likely this will occur by e-mail. The following characteristics should be considered in providing personal feedback to students:

- Multidimensional (covers content, presentation, and grammar);
- Nonevaluative (provides objective information);
- Supportive (offers information that will allow the learner to see areas for improvement);
- Receiver Controlled (allows the learner to accept or reject the information);
- Timely (provided as soon as possible after the intended work);
- Specific (precisely describes observations and recommendations)

The instructor should be sure to provide information at the beginning of class so that students know what is expected of them and what will be standard for evaluation and feedback. Instructor feedback should be clear, thorough, consistent, equitable, and professional. Since students require regular and constructive feedback from faculty, they will appreciate comments that indicate the instructor has tailored remarks for that particular individual.

Netiquette

Netiquette, or Internet etiquette, is a type of guideline for posting and sending messages in the online classroom. Netiquette not only covers rules of behavior but also guidelines for ensuring interaction in the online environment. Shea (2004) outlined core rules of netiquette that every online student should follow:

- Remember the human (never forget there is really a person behind the keystrokes);
- Adhere to the same standards of behavior online that you follow in real life (in other words, be ethical);
- Know where you are in cyberspace (i.e.; main discussion area, chat area);
- Respect each other's time and bandwidth (post appropriate messages);
- Make yourself look good online (check grammar and spelling);
- Share expert knowledge (help answer others' questions);
- Help keep tempers under control (don't respond to irate postings);
- Respect other people's privacy (do not read others private e-mail);
- Don't abuse your power;
- Be forgiving of other people's mistakes (you were once new to the online environment as well).

The core rules of netiquette were designed to help students who are new to the Internet to make friends instead of enemies. The instructor can post or link to these basic rules to help students understand the basic expectations of behavior online.

Special Considerations

Diversity and Americans with disabilities are global issues facing us daily as well as in the online environment. Since these issues are considered serious and sensitive to many people, instructors should consider human equity issues seriously.

Key Points on Diversity

Diversity consists of two dimensions, primary and secondary.

■ Primary dimensions are those characteristics that everyone is born with and that are visible and easy to identify. They include age, gender, race, ethnicity, and other physical characteristics.

■ Secondary dimensions are differences or characteristics that we acquire or change throughout our lives. These include work experience, income, marital status, religious beliefs, and education. These dimensions shape everyone we encounter in school, the workplace, and social settings. Valuing diversity according to the Center for Research on Education, Diversity and Excellence (2002) is:
   ■ Voluntary
   ■ Productivity driven
   ■ Qualitative
   ■ Opportunity focused
   ■ Proactive

Government agencies, corporations, and educational institutions are now recognizing the necessity of valuing diversity to remain competitive and effective. As a facilitator, one needs to eliminate stereotypes and become more educated about different groups. This way, one is less likely to generalize. Suggestions for doing this might include:

■ becoming aware of the stereotypes you hold;
■ determining the source of the stereotype and how it was formed;

- expanding your knowledge about other groups and cultures;
- expanding your experiences with other groups and cultures

Key points of Americans with Disabilities Act

Tulloch and Thompson (1999) identity security and testing issues in distance learning: They direct universities to make their distance learning classes accessible to qualified individuals with a disability, just as they are required to do for traditional courses. In particular, 42 U.S.C. sec. 12132 states:

> Subject to the provisions of this subchapter, no qualified individual with a disability shall, by reason of such disability, be excluded from participation in or be denied the benefits of the services, programs, or activities of a public entity, or be subjected to discrimination by any such entity.

For nonpublic institutions, 42 U.S.C. sec. 12182(a) provides:

> No individual shall be discriminated against on the basis of disability in the full and equal enjoyment of goods, services, privileges, advantages or accommodations of an entity.

As universities and faculty expand their distance-education offerings, they are finding that they must include the virtual equivalents of wheelchair ramps when building their online classrooms. They must accommodate, for instance, the student who is unable to see navigational graphics on a Web page because he is blind and the student who cannot listen to a streaming audio lecture because she is deaf. In fact, many students with disabilities find that Web site technological extravaganzas are more of a burden than an aid.

For the most part, distance-education students with disabilities already can get the equipment they need to make up for their impairments. Blind students can use software that reads online text aloud or produces a Braille message for the students to follow.

Students who cannot move their arms easily can use adaptive equipment to manipulate the computer with other parts of their bodies. But some common features of the Internet make navigation difficult for people with certain disabilities. Text-reading programs, for instance, are unable to recognize graphics. The problem is easily avoided if the programs can pick up and read aloud alternate texts that are placed behind the graphics, but not every Web site provides those texts. Sites with frames and tables (two commonly used features of Web page design) tend to confuse those programs, which often read from left to right, ignoring the layout. An important issue is for universities to determine exactly what the law requires.

As an online facilitator, the considerations for students with disabilities need to be taken on an individual basis. For example, if you know a student has a particular disability, you will need to take into account accommodations that may be necessary for this particular problem. It should be determined from the beginning exactly what the student's limitations are and what devices the student is using, if any; for example: TTY phones, screen readers, or voice recognition software. Allowing more time for test taking may be necessary for some individuals, or allowance for leniency on spelling if you know a student is using voice recognition software. If you are using audio files, for example, be sure to include a text version of the same information. If you are including Web references, be sure to check their format (amount of graphics, use of frames) for accommodating screen readers. *The bottom line is that everyone should have equal access to information.*

STUDENT ROLE

The student role in a distance course also changes significantly. Students must be more responsible for their own learning. There is greater emphasis on identifying one's own learning needs and making plans to achieve learning objectives (Billings, 1997). Prior to becoming an online student, the individual must have some basic knowledge of information technology in order to participate in a distance course. Gilbert (2001) suggests that students start by asking:

What is online learning and what is it like?

Where can I find it and is it for me?

What works in an online environment?

What criteria make a good candidate for online learning?

What are the advantages or disadvantages?

How do I choose an online learning provider?

How do I pick a curriculum?

How can I get information about sources?

What makes for a good distance program?

Where do I start?

How can I succeed?

How can I manage the tools and equipment?

When designing distance learning academic programs, the basic characteristics of students should be considered. Their age, interests, skill levels, academic preparedness, and career goals, for example, should be considered. Much of the literature suggests that older students and adults are the primary targets of distance programs. In the United States, typical adult distance-learning students are between the ages of twenty-five and fifty. Many online learners are adult students with family and job responsibilities who require the flexibility of online learning in order to advance in their job or to earn their degree. However, as more and more students become exposed to the online learning model, the traditional profile is changing.

So what criteria should the online student consider when doing a self-evaluation for distance learning? The Illinois Online Network (2008) suggests that the student possess the following qualities:

- *Students must be open minded and willing to share work, life, and educational experiences with fellow students in the classroom.* The online classroom should be and open and friendly environment.

- *Students should be able to communicate through writing.* Since nearly all online learning is written, it is important that student feel comfortable expressing themselves in writing.
- *Students must be motivated, self-disciplined and willing to "speak-up" if problems occur in the class.* The freedom and flexibility of the online classroom requires commitment and discipline for students to keep pace and requires communication with the instructor regarding any problems that may arise.
- *Students must be willing to commit to 4 to 15 hours per week of class hours per week per course.* Online is not easier than the traditional educational process. In fact, many students will say it requires much more time and commitment.
- *Students should accept critical thinking and be able to think ideas through before responding as part of the learning process.* The learning process requires the student to make decisions based on facts as well as experience. Assimilating information and executing the right decisions requires critical thought; case analysis does this very effectively.
- *Students must have access to a computer and a modem.* The student must have access to the necessary hardware and software requirements for participation in the course.
- *And finally, the students must feel that high quality learning can take place without going to a traditional classroom.* Online is not for everybody. A student who wants to be on a traditional campus attending a traditional classroom is probably not going to be satisfied with the online learning format. While the level of social interaction can be very high in the virtual classroom, it is not the same as living in a dorm on a campus with continuous opportunities for face to face social interaction. This should be made known. An online student is expected to:
  - Participate in the virtual classroom 3–5 out of 7 days a week
  - Be able to work with others in completing projects
  - Be able to use the technology properly
  - Be able to meet the minimum standards as set forth by the institution

- Be able to complete assignments on time
- Enjoy communicating in writing.

In your online course, you may want to include reference links to resources and tips for your students to use to help them be more successful online learners. Many universities have information on their home page that helps students with tips for success in online courses. Clearly outlining expectations and characteristics of a successful online student can help students determine if the online environment will be a productive learning environment for them. Often a questionnaire for prospective students to fill out to assess whether they are good candidates for online learning can be found on the university home page.

Student Expectations

Online students should expect that their instructor would provide the best learning environment possible. According to ION (2008) the student should expect that:

- The instructor will create the learning environment in such a way that learners can use their own experiences in the learning process and to translate theory to practice.
- The instructor should be concerned about the success of the learner, and every reasonable opportunity should be given to the learner to achieve.
- The instructor should give and solicit feedback. The feedback given by the instructor should keep the learner aware of his progress in the course. The feedback the instructor elicits from learners should guide the students' progress toward attaining objectives.
- The student should expect little or no lecturing.
- Tests that require memorization are least effective and case analysis would be more appropriate.
- The learner will be treated politely and respectfully.
- The instructor will provide contact information and days and times available.

With consistency in instructor delivery, students can anticipate and prepare their coursework based on expectations of how the instructor will run the course. When managing an online course, the faculty and the student play important roles. The faculty must plan for how the course will be managed based on student profiles, and the student must take responsibility for learning. A variety of characteristics including demographics, motivation, academic preparedness, and access to resources should be considered as important for an online learner.

In summary, course management covers a breadth of considerations, from student orientation, to discussion facilitation, to instructor feedback for students. It is interesting to note that each time an online course is taught, the instructor will note nuances or frequently asked questions that will help her prepare better for the next class. The students eventually will come armed with experience in online learning and will focus less on technology and management issues and more on course content.

Exhibit 8.1

SAMPLE OF AN ONLINE SYLLABUS

Course Syllabus

Course Number: xxxxxxxx

Course Title:

Course Start Date: xxxxxx

Course End Date: xxxxxx

Instructor—Your Name

Email Address: xxxxxxxx   Home Telephone Number: xxxxxxxx

Eastern Standard Time

Alternative/emergency e-mail address: xxxxxxxx

Instructor Availability: Indicate the best times and methods for students to reach you here.

Welcome class!

Provide a welcoming message and a brief bio on yourself.

General Course Description
This course develops the basic skills of critically analyzing research findings. Research methods are introduced with emphasis placed upon analyzing key elements of research reports.

Topics and Objectives: Provide a course overview here.

Class Biographies—Your first assignment is to post a biography in the main classroom using mine as a suggested format. Please feel free to use the chat area to respond to each other's bios and informally get to know each other.

Student materials

Books, Software, or Other Course Materials

List books required for the course here and a link to the university library

Electronic Resources: Provide relevant course links here.

Where to Go to Class—Your Class Meetings

Announcements
Assignments can be submitted to the digital drop box or to the instructors e-mail. Chat Room is designed as a place to discuss issues not related to the course content, but you can use it for discussion questions and things like that if you want.

Course Materials provide relevant documents for completing this course.

Group Work:
    Learning-Team A (List members)
    Learning-Team B
    Learning-Team C
    Learning-Team D

Technology Issues:
For problems with access into this course or other technology issues, please contact the University help desk or other designated location for online courses. Email: xxxxxxxx Phone Number: xxxxxxxx

APA and Attachments:
Some of your assignments require APA format. It is not possible to apply all the APA guidelines and have them transfer properly in OE notes, and so the University now requires that any assignments requiring APA format must be sent as attachments.
- Prepare these assignments in Microsoft Word.
- Save your work as a ".doc" file (this is the MS Word default file type).
- To send an attachment, open a "Reply Group" in the correct thread (or a new post if it is to the Assignments folder). Type in a subject line that includes the name of the assignment and your initials
- Use the "Attach" function to find and attach the file from your word processor.
- Then send it.

The Online Weekly Schedule: Please take note of the electronic weekly schedule. Remember that the week begins on Monday and ends on Sunday.

Day 1—Monday
Day 2—Tuesday
Day 3—Wednesday
Day 4—Thursday
Day 5—Friday
Day 6—Saturday
Day 7—Sunday

Administrative Issues

Course Changes—Although I will not make changes in the objectives of the course or change the course materials, I reserve the right to make slight modifications of the weekly assignments that vary from the curriculum as necessary

Attendance—In order to meet the university requirements for attendance, you must post at least one message to the course discussion board on two separate days during the online week. If you are out of attendance for one week or more of a class that is four weeks in length, or two or more weeks of a course that is five or more weeks, you will be automatically withdrawn and not be eligible to receive credit or earn a credit grade. (Please note: Check your university's policy on online attendance).

Participation—Class participation is different from attendance. I expect each student to contribute to the class in a substantive way on X out of seven days each week. By substantive, I mean postings that demonstrate thought and an attempt to discuss your personal work experiences, as they are relevant to the class discussion (approximately 100–150 words). I will not be counting participation in the study group area as class participation. Please remember that I am looking for quality, not necessarily quantity.

Late Assignments—Late assignments will be downgraded by one point for each day that they are late. An assignment is considered late if it is posted after midnight your time zone on the day it is due. If unforeseen circumstances prohibit you from turning in an assignment on time, be sure to contact me to negotiate for an alternative submission date.

Writing Assignments—All papers must adhere to the university writing style guidelines (Little, Brown Compact Handbook or APA Manual). Written assignments must include a cover page, abstract, and references. Your written work is a representation of you. Insure all credits are given for other's work. Any violations, plagiarism, or copying will not be tolerated. *Please also ensure all written assignments have a defined summary at the end of the paper.

Incomplete Grades—I do not grant "incompletes" in my class. Therefore it is imperative that you submit all final graded requirements by their due date.

Weekly Summary—Each week you will present a brief (250 words or less) weekly summary that summarizes what you learned from the readings, research, activities, and assignments. This summary is due at the end of each week. Please include two paragraphs summarizing (1) what you learned from the course materials and (2) what you learned from your classmates. Students are not expected to present a weekly summary for the final week of the course.

Group Work—Learning teams (or groups) will be developed on Sunday during the first week of class. You will be asked to participate in one of these groups (group A, B, C, or D). I will be assigning you to a group based on backgrounds and experience. GROUP WORK—you will receive your first group assignment on xxxxxxx. You will then work with this group for the remainder of the course. Your grade for your group work will be the same for all group members. Your group project final postings will be in the MAIN Classroom so that you can share your final product with your classmates. Please feel free to contact me if you feel strongly about working with a particular individual in your group or if any problems arise. (Some people prefer to work together by time zones or work schedules). Just remember, all work is asynchronous so we should accommodate everyone!

Academic Honesty

Academic honesty is highly valued online just as it is at each University setting. A student must always submit work that represents his or her original words or ideas. If any words or ideas are used that do not represent the student's original words or ideas, the student must cite all relevant sources. The student should also make clear the extent to which such sources were used. Words or ideas that require citations include, but are not limited to, all hard copy or electronic publications, whether copyrighted or not, and all verbal or visual communication when the content of such communication clearly originates from an identifiable source. At the online campus, all submissions to any public meeting site or private mailbox fall within the scope of words and ideas that require citations if used by someone other than the original author.

Academic dishonesty in an online learning environment includes:

- Having a tutor or friend complete a portion of your assignments;
- Having a reviewer make extensive revisions to an assignment;
- Copying work submitted by another student to a public class meeting;
- Using information from online information services without proper citation.

Grading Formula—I will not round grades numerically (either up or down) when it comes to graded papers and projects. I will not round on final grades. For example, final grade of 89.9% will be considered a B; however, other factors, such as the quality of your participation, will be considered.

Your overall class participation grade is based upon your general comments and interactions in all the forums, your Discussion Question inputs to the Main Forum, and your weekly overviews. You will get a chance to submit your own answers to the Discussion Questions as well as selectively comment on the submissions of interest made by other students. I will assign a participation grade each week (based on your general comments and overall interactions). Your Discussion Question responses the timeliness and quality of your comments to other student Discussion Questions and your weekly overviews will be graded appropriately. I will give you weekly feedback using points to let you know how you are doing. For example, if you provide great answers to the discussion questions, participate actively and thoughtfully in the discussions, and demonstrate what you have learned in your weekly summary, then you will have earned your full three points for the week!!

Grading
A+ 94–100
A 90–93
A- 87–89
B+ 83–86

POINT VALUES FOR THE COURSE

Assignments	*Percent*
Individual (70%)	10
Paper One (Due end of week One)	
Paper Two (Due end of week Two)	10
Paper Three (Due end of week Three)	10
Paper Four (Due end of week Four)	15
Paper Five (Due end of week Five)	15
Participation (Weekly)	10
Learning Team (30%)	15
Presentation One (Due end of week Four)	
Presentation (Due end of week Five)	15
Total	**100**

Include Course Schedule Here:

REFERENCES

ADA Home Page. (2008). Americans with Disabilities. Retrieved April 22, 2008, from http://www.ada.gov

Billings, D. (1997). Issues in teaching and learning at a distance: Changing roles and responsibilities of administrators, faculty and students. *Computers in Nursing*, 15(2), 69–70.

Center for Research on Education, Diversity, and Excellence. (2002). Retrieved April 22, 2008, from http://www.crede.ucsc.edu

Gilbert, S. (2001). *How to be a successful online student*. New York: McGraw-Hill.

Illinois Online Network (2008). Retrieved April 22, 2008, from http://www.ion.uillinois.edu/resources

Kimball, L. (2002). Managing distance learning—new challenges for faculty. Retrieved April 28, 2008, from http://www.stratfordhigh.school.nz/home/jr/readings/teaching_under_the_microscope.pdf

Palloff, R. & Pratt, K. (1999). *Building learning communities in cyberspace: Effective strategies for the online classroom*. San Francisco: Jossey-Bass Publishers.

Perrin, D. (1999). The level of interactivity on the Internet and the Web. Retrieved January 20, 1999, from http://usdla.org/html/journal/ APR99_Issue/16_ed_apr_99c.htm

Ryan, M., Hodson-Carlton, K., & Ali, N. (2005). A model for faculty teaching online: Confirmation of a dimensional matrix. *Journal of Nursing Education*, 44(8), 357–364.

Shea, V. (2004). Net Etiquette. Retrieved April 22, 2008, from http://www.albion.com/netiquette/introduction.html

Assessment and Evaluation of Online Learning

CAROL A. O'NEIL AND CHERYL A. FISHER

Assessing the learner involves gathering data to identify needs, ability, and progress. Assessment is student-oriented and is used to place, promote, graduate, or retain students. Evaluation is a judgment made by comparing a behavior to a standard. Evaluation is the measurement of a behavior and the comparison of that behavior to a predetermined expectation.

ASSESSMENT, EVALUATION, AND PEDAGOGY

Pedagogical theory forms the framework for the design of a learning experience. Learning objectives, learning strategies, and evaluation activities flow from the pedagogical theory. For example, if an instructor uses behavioral theory to design a learning experience, you would expect to see learning objectives that focus on the targeted behavior and strategies that include rewards and consequences. The objectives and strategies drive the evaluation activities. If the learning objective is to state five signs and symptoms of congestive heart failure, the evaluation should measure whether the learner can state the signs and symptoms. To determine if the student has achieved this objective, the student may be asked to name the five signs and symptoms or may be asked to answer a multiple-choice question related to the topic.

TRADITIONAL ASSESSMENT AND EVALUATION

A traditional evaluation design measures the attainment of learning objectives through exams, papers, and projects that the student submits to the instructor. The instructor uses criteria to grade the student's assignments and to categorize them into a grade of "A," "B," and so forth. The student demonstrates learning as stipulated in the objectives, and based on the degree of attainment of those objectives, a grade is assigned. This is called norm-referenced assessment, because we make judgments about learning and a bell-shaped curve is an expected outcome. This means that some students get grades of D or F, others get A grades, and the mean is about a B or C. The students are responsible for their learning and their grade. Another type of assessment is criterion-referenced, which is based on learning for the purpose of meeting a standard. In this type of assessment, the instructor is responsible for helping all learners meet the standard. An example of a standard is validation, such as CPR validation.

In addition to the students, traditional evaluation includes gathering data about the course from an end-of-course survey that is completed by students. An administrator compiles the data, and sometime after the end of the course, gives the results to the faculty to review. Data may be used to make changes in the course delivery before the next time it is offered.

Traditional assessments may also include measuring the students' progress through a course or on the way to completing the course. Usually assessment techniques are process oriented and might take the form of a quiz. The purpose of assessment is to check the progress of students to identify those who may be struggling through the course.

CONSTRUCTIVISM AND ONLINE LEARNING

When constructivism is the guiding theory in learning, students construct new knowledge by actively engaging in learning strategies. Students reflect on the learned content and their reflections bring meaning to a larger social context or solve real world problems. Learning is process oriented, and when basic knowledge is used to construct new knowledge, the basic knowledge is reinforced. Traditional evaluation designs that predominantly focus on measuring the students' learning of objectives will not provide a comprehensive picture of the students' learning. Focusing on the students' learning processes while they are constructing new knowledge is important. While learners are constructing new knowledge, they need feedback. Feedback means that learners need comments from teachers that will motivate them to continue constructing knowledge or to continue moving in a constructive direction.

A traditional evaluation design does not accommodate the use of technology as a learning tool. Let us say that a student registers for a fully Web-based course and shows up at the faculty's office the second week of the semester asking where the class will be held. Somehow, the student already has missed information and thus progress is hampered. By the second week of the semester, the student should have the computer skills needed to negotiate the online course, should have the needed resources (i.e., course entry information such as user name and password), and should know how to navigate through the course. If the student does not have these basic skills, the student will have to spend time learning navigational skills instead of course material. To get the student directly into the learning material, precourse student assessments should be planned into the design of the learning experiences.

These assessments should provide data about the student's readiness to take a course online. Data gathered about the student's readiness should be summarized and a prescriptive plan should be developed that will guide the learner to resources needed to be successful online. The prescriptive plan is written and individualized for each student. The plan includes activities and outcomes that focus on the skills that will ensure success online. Some examples include: knowing how to download files, navigating the Web, receiving and sending e-mail, sending attachments, and basic typing skills.

When developing learning material online, the learning material should be peer reviewed before it is released to learners. A peer review is a process in which a designated reviewer uses established criteria to review a course.

Information gathered from the review is shared with the course developers so corrections can be made before students log on to the course. A peer review is crucial for newly developed courses, because there may be links that do not work, there may be spelling and grammatical errors, or there may be exam dates in the syllabus that are not the same as the dates on a calendar. The purpose of a peer review is to enhance the quality of learning.

The reviewer has a "fresh set of eyes" that can detect glaring errors so they can be corrected before the learners arrive. It is recommended that peers review or follow a course while it is offered to students. Faculty should be recognized for their contributions and successes when they teach online. Faculty who teach online should ask content and technology experts to "sit-in" on their courses as guests to provide feedback for the faculty. The feedback can be used for tenure and promotion, to promote recognition of scholarship of teaching and learning online, and to provide visibility for online courses especially to faculty who do not teach online.

Technology has influences on the course before it is offered, while it is being offered, and at the end of the course. Online learners need an orientation to the technology and learning platform before the course starts. Evaluating the effectiveness of the orientation is important for revising and refining. During the course, servers can crash and hard drives can go down. For example, during one semester, students were assigned to gather secondary data about a community. Data about the behavioral indicators of a community, such as smoking, obesity, prenatal care, and so forth, which were located on a server that was managed by the state health department. About a week before starting content on the community assessment module, the information was pulled offline by the state health department. The faculty checked the links to this Web site before the course started, so the faculty did not know the link was not working when the students were working on the assignment. But the students knew and the e-mails from students to faculty increased.

Evaluating the online course while it is live is essential. Early in the course, the faculty can ask students to e-mail them with anything that looks like a course issue as soon as it becomes apparent. Give students permission to ask "dumb" questions like "Should the syllabus icon go to the syllabus?" Faculty needs information to quickly correct whatever glitches may arise. Aside from technical issues, there could be learner issues. Conflicts between students may develop or there could be hurt feelings because someone typed something that someone else read as negative. A quick response to technical and student issues while the course is running prevents further (and usually more chaotic) repercussions. At the end, the course needs to be evaluated by faculty, learners, and instructional designers using tools that focus on gathering data that is particular to online courses.

Summary of Traditional vs. Online Assessment and Evaluation

In summary, evaluation of online learning differs from that of traditional classroom learning. Assessing the learner is an essential component in online learning. Learners' skills and ability need to be assessed, learners' responses to orientation needs to be assessed, learners need feedback during the course while they are constructing new knowledge, and learners need grades assigned at the end of the course. Therefore, traditional assessment and evaluation models need to be revised to accommodate learning online.

FOUNDATIONAL KNOWLEDGE ON ASSESSMENT AND EVALUATION

The Committee on the Foundations of Assessment (Pellegrino, Ludowsky, Glasser, 2001) depicts the foundational knowledge on assessment and evaluation as a triangle with three key elements: cognition, observation, and interpretation. These three elements are connected to and dependent on each other. Cognition is defined as the aspects of achievement that will be assessed. Observation is the collecting of evidence about the students' achievement. Interpretation is the methodology used to analyze the collected evidence.

Smith and Ragan (1999) use the term "evaluation." They offer two purposes of evaluation: to assess individual student's performances and to provide information to revise course material. Smith and Ragan call evaluation a way of "getting there:" Did the student "get there" and how well did the instruction get the student there. They suggest that assessments be based on the learning objectives, and these are called criterion-referenced assessment items. Their purpose is to assess competence or to identify gaps in learning, but they do not compare or rank learners. That is the purpose of norm-referenced tests. Smith and Ragan write that assessments are either criterion or norm referenced, thus alluding to two types of assessment: to identify gaps and to compare students' learning.

They describe three types of assessments: entry skills assessments, preassessments, and postassessments. The entry skills assessment focuses on skills needed to be successful in the online course; preassessments focus on ascertaining what the students already know, and postassessments focus on attainment of learning objectives. They outline characteristics of good assessment instruments as: validity, reliability, and practicality. A valid assessment answers the question: Does it measure what it claims it will measure? A reliable instrument is one that yields consistent outcomes over time. A practical assessment is cost effective. Smith and Ragan (1999) suggest two formats of assessment: performance assessment and paper-and-pencil tests.

Smith and Ragan (1999) further describe evaluation as a means of providing information to revise course material and offer two types of evaluation: formative and summative. Formative evaluations provide information for the purpose of revising the instruction, and summative evaluations provide data about the continued use of the instruction.

NEW MODEL FOR ASSESSING AND EVALUATING ONLINE LEARNING

The authors of this book developed a model that incorporates the foundations of assessment and evaluation, guided constructivism, and online learning. The following questions were asked: Did the teaching methods and strategies used in this learning experience effectively impart information? Did the recipients learn the information? These questions are answered when assessing student learning and evaluating the course.

Assessment and evaluation are activities that are planned when the course is designed. The activities should be appropriate and congruous measures of the goals and objectives of the course. The activities provide data that can be used to make judgments about student learning and course effectiveness. Data can be gathered about the feasibility of student success online, the progress of the student through the course, student achievement of the course objectives at the end of the course, the effectiveness of the course design, the effectiveness of the course while it is taught, and the outcomes of the course. Student learning and course functioning are two aspects that need to be addressed separately. A model is suggested that will focus on student learning and course evaluations separately.

Assessment focuses on the student, and evaluation focuses on the course. Assessment and evaluation are built into the course design and are visible throughout the course from even before the beginning to after the course ends.

Assessment is defined as the identification of student needs and progress throughout the learning experience. The purpose of precourse assessments is to identify the needs of the student so they can be remediated before the course begins. During the course, the focus is on the students' progress. The faculty monitors the students throughout the course and gives feedback about the process of constructing new knowledge. Assessing the learner at the end of the course is determined by graded activities. Grading criteria should be clearly specified in the syllabus.

Evaluation focuses on the course itself. Precourse evaluation includes peer review of the course and an evaluation of the orientation program that is given to students before they enter the course. Formative evaluation is directed at how the course is operating, and summative evaluation is evaluation of the course after it is completed.

A new model called The Model for Assessing and Evaluating Learning Online, as seen in Figure 9.1, was developed based on

Student Assessment

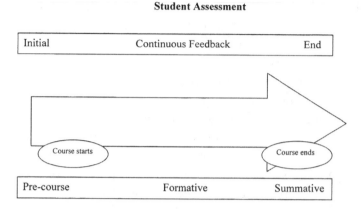

Course Evaluation

Figure 9.1 The model for assessing and evaluating learning online.

Smith and Ragan (1999). The aspects of achievement are divided into three phases for student assessment and three phases of course evaluation.

During each phase, evidence is gathered and analyzed. At each phase decisions are made based on the analyzed evidence. For example, at the end of the initial phase of student assessment, a prescriptive plan is developed which outlines knowledge and competencies that the student needs to master to continue in the course. During the continuous assessment, students are given feedback and motivation to help them determine their progress. The end student assessment is the measure of individual achievement. Evidence is gathered about the student's ability to meet objectives, and a decision to pass or fail is determined.

Student Initial Assessment

Researchers have identified various types of initial student assessment techniques. Faculty and course developers can use these techniques to determine a range of student skills from comfort with technology to preferred learning styles. The following list includes some suggestions for faculty to use when conducting an initial student assessment prior to participating in an online course:

- Initial letter of assessment about the student as a learner;
- Placement exams;
- Students develop personal Web pages;
- Electronic meeting;
- Computer skills exercise;
- Pretests;
- Scavenger hunt to assess navigation skills, (develop a scavenger hunt list and posting of announcements; ask students to find the items and e-mail the answers to the instructor);
- Learning style surveys;
- Readiness surveys;
- Continuous feedback.

Continuous student feedback can be conducted at any time during the course. The purpose of continuous feedback is to determine if the student is learning from the course material presented. It is important for the faculty to know if the lectures and content of the course have been presented in a clear and logical format. Obtaining this information prior to the end of the course enables the instructor to make changes. Some of these techniques include:

- Journaling, writing marathons, diaries: techniques to assess attitude and satisfaction (affective objectives);
- Creating written logs about experiences and reflections;
- Concept mapping: connective key concepts;
- Giving midsemester assessment;
- Estimating student time ranges for each assignment plus interaction;
- Giving feedback;
- Having three-minute "things I don't understand about" sessions;
- Assigning a weekly new idea;
- Debating;
- Asking students to answer the question: What was the fuzziest point?
- Assigning reaction paper;
- Assigning worksheets;

- Giving nongraded quizzes;
- Using simulations;
- Assigning crossword puzzles;
- Tracking attendance;
- Allowing peer questions to other students;
- Encouraging participation in discussion board;
- Assigning homework;
- Questioning;
- Assigning case studies: detailed accounts of a client, family, group (pregnant teens); or community;
- Completing a student assessment.

At the end of a course, students are assessed in terms of meeting the course learning objectives. Multiple methods can be used and the following list identifies some methods:

- Quizzes;
- Compositions, essays, and papers;
- Projects (individual or group); project summaries, Web-page presentations;
- Analysis of newspaper article;
- Examinations: exams can be multiple choice and/or essay. Exams can be timed and proctored to ensure that students submit their own work. Students can take exams in schools of nursing, at outreach sites, at community colleges with faculty proctors, at local libraries, or at home with approved proctors. Exams can be proctored at testing centers such as the Sylvan Learning Centers. Proctoring by video may also be an option.
- Portfolios: (e-folios), which are collections of student work in the course stored in a digital medium such as a CD. The work may include reflective essays, patient care plans, pamphlets developed for a health fair, pictures of a health project at an immunization fair, or an audiotape of a song to prevent teen pregnancy.
- Student presentations;
- Peer evaluation;

- Final interviews;
- Rubrics.

Rubrics are sets of standards that can be used to assign grades and give students feedback about their performance. Rubrics can use descriptions or commentaries on achievement, such as excellent, good, fair, or poor. They can be based on competencies, and they can address multidimensional skills such as a group project (Huba & Freed, 2000). Anderson, Bauer, and Speck (2002) provide examples of rubrics that can be used to assess student work in chat rooms, bulletin boards, on written or group projects, and in-field experiences. An abbreviated rubric for assessing chat room participation (Anderson, Bauer & Speck, 2002, p. 33) is:

9–10 points for logging into chat room on time and fully participating in discussions

7–8 points for logging in with variable participation in discussions

5–6 points for logging in late and participating infrequently in discussions

1–4 points for missing chats and rarely participating in discussions

Precourse Evaluation

Precourse evaluation helps faculty to determine if the course is ready for launching. An external, objective reviewer should ideally review the course for content and for instructional design. The peer reviewer should then continue to observe the course for interaction approximately two weeks into the course and again at midterm. The reviewer should provide constructive feedback to the instructor, which can be used to make changes in the course. Preevaluation activities can include:

- Peer review of content
- Peer review of design

Table 9.1

CRITERIA FOR PEER REVIEW OF ONLINE COURSES*

THE WEB COURSE PROFILING CATEGORIES
PART ONE: REVIEW OF THE COURSE DESIGN AND IMPLEMENTATION

1. Course rationale and syllabus
2. Goals and objectives
3. Instructional design for Web environments
4. Theoretical basis for learning and teaching (pedagogical foundations)
5. Content and metacontent
6. Learning and teaching strategies and activities
7. Interactivity and community building (with faculty, students, and content)
8. Use of mediated resources, electronic libraries, and the Web
9. Orientation, induction into online learning, metalearning (learning how to learn online)
10. Responsiveness to learner needs (learning-centric, learner sensitive)
11. Diversity, multiple cultural perspectives, accommodation for geographic distance
12. Assessment and evaluation
13. Accessibility, robustness, and technical support (infrastructure and ease of use for instructor and students)
14. Interface design and navigation
15. Intellectual property: copyright, attribution, rights for use
16. Internal organization and consistency (Overriding Criteria)

PART TWO: REVIEW OF PILOT DELIVERY AND TEACHING EFFECTIVENESS

1. Instructor's role and teaching effectiveness
2. Students' levels of engagement, motivation, achievement, and satisfaction

- Ongoing peer review
- Course review by students
- Evaluation of orientation to online learning

Fellows in the Web Initiative in Teaching Project (WIT, a University System of Maryland faculty initiative, 1998–2002) developed a Peer Review Process for new online courses. Margaret Chambers, Director of the Institute of Distance Education at the University of Maryland University College and the Web Initiative in Teaching Project, wrote the letter found in Exhibit 9.1 to external peer reviewers to describe the peer review process. The peer review criteria can be found in Table 9.1.

FORMATIVE EVALUATION

Formative evaluation throughout the course allows the faculty to determine if course delivery, structure, or instructional design needs revising. For example, students may ask for a discussion forum to list technology issues and ask for peer help. By providing students with the opportunity to ask questions during the course, issues can be resolved quickly and students can focus on their learning. Some suggestions for formative evaluation are:

- "Pulse Check:" ask students on a regular basis, maybe every four weeks or three times during the semester, to post or email their "pulse"—where they are and how they are doing in the course, and what improvements or changes they think should be made;
- Discussion summaries every other week about course content and issues;
- Midsemester survey;
- Verbal feedback to specific questions;
- Summative Evaluation: the institution often requires summative evaluation. This evaluation provides feedback to the faculty to revise the course and to evaluate the faculty. Examples include:
    - Student evaluation of course
    - Student evaluation of faculty
    - Faculty evaluation of course

The Web Initiative in Teaching Fellows in the WIT Project developed a pool of questions based on the categories of an effective online course. They developed questions for three audiences: the reviewer, the instructor, and the student. You can use this pool by first choosing your audience. If you are developing a survey for students as an end-of-course survey, look in the student column of the Pool of Potential Items in Appendix A, found on pages 153–163 in the first edition. Read the items and choose the ones that are reflective and pertinent to your student population. Including items from each category will enhance the validity of the survey.

Exhibit 9.1

The WIT peer review process was developed in response to concerns of tenure track faculty who wish to receive recognition for the scholarship of teaching that is needed to create and teach a successful Web-based course. Throughout the developmental process we have engaged in peer feedback using an evolving set of criteria or profiling characteristics (see the bottom of this message). This external review of the teaching pilot is intended to ascertain the overall quality of the Web course to facilitate active learning and interaction. Each WIT external peer review committee will consist of two discipline specialists and will be coordinated by a WIT Fellow from another institution who successfully authored and taught a Web-based course the previous year.

Each peer review committee will receive a set of review questions based on the profiling categories and will be asked to complete two questionnaires, one in early October and the other at the end of the semester. By the end of January, the team will be asked to submit a brief narrative report(s) based upon the review questions/categories. Unlike a face-to-face classroom, the Web-enabled virtual classroom is open for your observations throughout the semester at your convenience. We are asking that you make an initial visit to the course Web site at the beginning of the semester, acquainting yourself with the syllabus and structure of the course, visiting the interactive conferencing, and testing the ease and logic of navigation around the Web course site. We will send you an electronic questionnaire the third week in September to gather your initial observations.

Asynchronous discussions unfold over time. We would like to have you visit the course for an entire week at least once in order to observe the pacing and style of learning interactions. An alternative might be to select and follow a module from the beginning to the end. Some of you may "shadow" the course on a weekly basis throughout the semester. The key is that you observe sufficiently to get an accurate reading of the quality of the interaction between the instructor and the students, and among the students.

Your final questionnaire will be sent around Thanksgiving and will be due by December 15. A short narrative report from the team as a whole or from individuals will be due by January 15.

You will receive instructions on how to access your Web course immediately from the course instructor. We hope you will find this experience broadens your knowledge and appreciation of teaching on the Web. On behalf of all the WIT Project participants, I want to thank you for your willingness to participate in this undertaking.

Margaret Chambers
Director

California State University–Chico's (2002) Committee for Evaluation of Exemplary Online Courses has developed a rubric to identify a quality online course. The criteria include: online organization and design, instructional design and delivery, assessment and evaluation of student learning, appropriate and effective use of technology, and learner support and resources. Baseline, effective, and exemplary quality are delineated.

In summary, a model has been developed that can be used to assess student learning and evaluate the learning environment. It incorporates the foundations of assessment and evaluation, guided constructivism, and online learning. Students should be assessed before the course starts to determine needs and learning style, during the course to determine progress, and at the end of the course as a final assessment of attaining goals. The course is peer evaluated before it is opened to students. Frequent evaluation of the course while it is being offered helps to identify problems and issues that can be remedied. Evaluating the course at the end provides data to revise the course and data that can be used in developing new courses.

REFERENCES

Anderson, R. S., Bauer, J. F., & Speck, B. W. (2002). *Assessment strategies for the on-line class: From theory to practice.* San Francisco: Jossey-Bass.

California State University–Chico. (n.d.). Rubric for online instruction. Retrieved April 2, 2008, from http://www.csuchico.edu/celt/roi/index.shtml

Huba, M. E. & Freed, J. E. (2000). *Learner-centered assessment on college campuses: Shifting the focus from teaching to learning.* Boston: Allen and Bacon Publishers.

Pellegrino J. W., Chudowsky, N., Glasser, R. (2001). Knowing What Students Know: The science and design of educational assessment. Retrieved April 2, 2008, from http://www.nap.edu/catalog.php?record_id=10019#toc

Smith, P. & Ragan, T. (2005). *Instructional Design* (3rd ed.). New York: John Wiley & Sons, Inc.

10 Distance and Continuing Medical Education

WILLIAM A. SADERA AND CHERYL A. FISHER

The availability of technology-supported Continuing Education (CE) for medical professionals began emerging in the early 1990's (Casebeer, Kristofco, Strasser, Reilly, Krishnamoorthy, Rabin, Zheng, Karp, & Myers, 2004). Since this time, physicians, nurses, and other health care professionals have continued to seek available technology-supported CE because of its convenience and accessibility. A recent review of online CE offerings showed that the number of sites had risen from 5% to 18% between 2003 and 2006 (Sklar, 2006); CME Web (the largest source for online CE), accredited by the American Academy of Continuing Medical Education (ACCME), offers 885 courses and over 800 hours of credit annually.

Telecommunications and distance-learning technologies are not new, but increased capabilities and the potential to reach a larger audience have transformed how we deliver education and training. More importantly, it has expanded our capacity to respond to the need to keep health professionals' knowledge and experiences current. With a long history of serving isolated and remote learners, distance learning has now emerged as an effective, mainstream delivery method of education and training that provides flexible learning opportunities in response to the needs of learners.

Over the past 15 to 20 years, research has helped us to understand the status and quality of distance-based teaching and learning in CE (Davis, O'Brien, & Freemantle, 1999; Fox 1991). However, the results of these studies have often been ignored and the results have not been applied to new course design. Although the findings of these studies are essential to the quality of the learning opportunities, administrators and faculty have not effectively adopted and integrated the findings to improve current course design and subsequent improved course outcomes. The result of not integrating research into practice has led to the disintegration of CE course quality.

This chapter will provide an overview of current issues related to the growth in use of online learning in CE. Because the research evidence was not applied, yet the demand continued to grow, CE courses were mass-produced without thoughtful application of sound pedagogical design. The purpose of this chapter is to review the current best practices and discuss the application of sound pedagogy and effective design. Finally, this chapter will culminate in a proposed model for integration of best practices and pedagogy that can be used to design future CE learning environments.

ISSUES FACING DISTANCE-BASED CE

Three issues confront distance based CE today. The first is the rapid expansion of CE offerings, second is the lack of pedagogical design, and third is the lack of integration of emerging technologies to facilitate design aspects of the learning environment. Pressures from the growing nursing shortage and state and regulatory requirements for CE and continuing education credit (CEU) credits led to institutions offering significantly more courses than they ever had in the past. Heller, Oros and Durney-Crowley (2003) noted that distance-based nursing has seen a rapid expansion of online course offerings, including entire Registered Nurse (RN) to Bachelor of Science in Nursing (BSN) curricula due to both the nursing shortage and the accompanying nursing faculty shortage. Additionally, this learning format is well suited to these working adults who benefit from the convenience of technology-supported continuing education as active working professionals. Given these factors, combined with the convenience and flexibility afforded through online education, offerings in this format will only continue to increase. However, along with the increasing demand and growing consumer experience with distance learning modalities, expectations for quality instruction, successful educational outcomes, and satisfying learning experiences will also increase (DeBourgh, 2001).

Fox (1991) noted that institutions have sacrificed the application of research findings to improve CE design at the expense of demand for quantity as opposed to quality. CE developers must implement strategies to effectively integrate pedagogical principles in order to return quality to CE learning opportunities.

In addition to concerns regarding the integration of sound pedagogical principles, most CE has not been rigorously evaluated; few courses are based on sound educational principles, and most do not employ strategies to optimize the learning opportunities afforded by new learning technologies (Casebeer, et al. 2004; Zimitat, 2001). This issue is compounded by the fact that CE is intertwined with the future of medical practice and the expansion in scientific knowledge, increasingly sophisticated diagnostic technologies, and the evolving complexity of clinical practice (Abrahamson, Baron, Elstein, Hammond, Holzman, Marlow, Taggart, & Shulkin, 1999). The success of technology-supported CE is threatened by inadequate quality assurance and a lack of careful educational design (Keane, Norman & Vickers, 1991). Additionally, most offerings do not make use of the unique ability of the technology to offer multiple paths for learning new material, nor do they take advantage of the technologies' capacities to support interactive student participation (Sklar, 2006).

As technology advances and CE expands in the direction of distance based courses, online CE providers need to research and continually assess learning within these environments. In a review of 30 CE courses, quality of content was the characteristic most important to participants, and too little interaction was the largest source of dissatisfaction (Casebeer, et al., 2004). Cobb (2004) reported on nine distance CE studies that found that the distance format was effective in imparting new knowledge and three studies that found that distance methods were effective but not superior. One study found that case-based distance courses were more effective than text-based formats. The authors suggested that increased satisfaction with this format may have been due to the interactive strategies that were employed (Casebeer et al., 2004). This research shows that distance CE can be effective, but it is the design of these courses that needs to be carefully scrutinized to ensure a successful learning experience. The CE developers are responsible to respond to the needs of the professionals to design, deliver, and evaluate new approaches to course design in order to determine the effectiveness of meeting the required outcomes.

PEDAGOGY AND CONTINUING EDUCATION

Because the primary audience for CE comprises working adult learners, ideally, institutions should show consideration for these learners so that they have a choice in the organization and delivery of the learning program. During their careers, these professionals need a range of topics in continuing education to enhance their clinical skills and knowledge while providing care to patients. Specifically, the aim of most CE is to help improve practices and behaviors in order to provide the best quality care to patients and to maintain currency in practice. Nurses specifically require CE for acquiring new knowledge, skills, and attitudes that must be learned in order to keep pace with changes in the field. Traditional continuing professional education is taught through passive activities, such as lectures, practical classes, and seminars. This kind of professional education usually requires the participants to be in the same place at the same time, which often does not coincide with the time demands of the three-shift work schedules.

Schools have traditionally provided CE through media such as lectures, audio and videotapes, and printed monographs. Over the years, similar distance learning technologies and methods have been applied to the continuing medical education needs for rural and remote physicians. They have included audio teleconferencing, correspondence study, and compressed videoconferencing. But providers have not adapted the instructional strategies to meet the capabilities of the technology or the learners. The recent emergence and growth of the Internet, World Wide Web, and compact disc read-only-memory (CD-ROM) technologies have introduced new opportunities for providing continuing education into the mainstream of health professionals (Curran, 2005) and the opportunity for new types of learning experiences to occur.

ADULT LEARNING AND CONTINUING EDUCATION

Part of being an effective instructor involves understanding how your learners learn. Adults, compared to children and teens, have distinct needs and requirements as learners. It should be noted that adult learning is not a unique and specific process. Instead generalizations about "the adult learner" imply that people over a certain, yet to be defined age form a homogenous group. However, differences of culture, cognitive style, life experiences, and gender may be far more important to learning than age (Shannon, 2003).

Adult learners are autonomous and self-directed (Knowles, 1970). Their teachers must actively involve adult participants in the learning process and serve as facilitators for them. Instructors should allow the participants to assume responsibility for presentations and group leadership. They must purposefully act as facilitators, guiding participants to their own knowledge rather than supplying them with facts. Adult learners have accumulated a foundation of life experiences and knowledge that may include work-related activities, family responsibilities, and previous education (Knowles, 1970). They need, then, to connect learning to this knowledge and experience base. To help these learners do so, instructors should draw out participants' experience and knowledge. Educators must relate theories and concepts to the participants and recognize the value of experience in learning. Additionally, instructors should treat these adults as equals in experience and knowledge and allow them to voice their opinions freely in class (Knowles, 1970). Because of these characteristics, adult-learning programs should capitalize on the experience of the participants and they should adapt to the age range of the participants. The course offerings should also provide as much choice as possible in the organization of the learning program.

SOCIAL INTERACTION AND CE

Social interaction has long been thought to increase collaboration and therefore result in increased learning. One research study found that a group participating in social interaction was more satisfied and performed better on outcome measures (Jung, Choi, Lim, & Leem, 2002). In this study, the collaborative interaction group expressed the highest level of satisfaction with their learning experience, and the collaborative and social interaction groups participated more actively in posting their opinions than the academic interaction group. The conclusions of this study are in line with the aforementioned needs of the adult learner.

Interaction has less to do with personal interaction (e.g., building a community of learners) and more to do with providing a means of reinforcing various elements from the content of the training (Giguere, Formica, and Harding, 2004). This interaction has been recognized as one of the most important components of learning experiences both in conventional education (Vygotsky, 1978) and distance education (Moore, 1993). Research has shown that learning in groups improves students' achievement of learning objectives. Vygotsky believes that cognitive development and learning are dependent on social interaction. The major theme of his theoretical framework is that social interaction plays a fundamental role in the process of learning.

A second aspect of Vygotsky's theory is the idea that the potential for cognitive development is limited to a certain "time span," which he refers to as the zone of proximal development (ZPD). It is during this time that consciousness is raised and a range of skills can be developed with adult guidance or peer collaboration. Vygotsky's methods of analysis and conclusions about the development of human thought and language are still regarded today and can be applied to the study of computer mediated communication (Bacalarski, n.d.). Given the interactive nature of online learning environments and the needs of

adult learners, the connections between these theories and this population is self-evident.

KEY PEDAGOGICAL CONSIDERATION

We have noted several key pedagogical considerations as repeat
themes in the distance-learning and continuing education literature.
These include accessibility and learner preference, interaction, and
quality of the course design. The following section of this chapter will
address these issues.

Accessibility and Learner Preferences

Dolcourt, Zuckerman, and Warner (2006) noted competing time
demands, irrelevant topics, and inconveniences such as parking and
inclement weather as major factors for poor attendance at CE educational offerings in traditional formats. Improved accessibility, afford-
ability of distance education, and time efficiency compared to the
traditional conference type programs are often cited as the primary
reasons for offering distance CE (Piemme, 2000). Piemme suggests
that CE providers are well-aware of the professional's busy schedule
and are trying to accommodate their needs by offering ease of access
and time efficiency. As consumers of educational products, busy healthcare providers make choices among competing alternatives for their
time. By recognizing key decision factors, CE developers can poten-
tially increase attendance and satisfaction by structuring style, content,
and logistics to better accommodate the learners' perspectives.

Although distance education programs enhance access to CE for the
health professional, increased access is often coupled with decreased
quality in course design. According to Carriere and Harvey (2001),
good course quality must take into consideration an understanding of
the experiences of the providers. As a result of this need for understanding, a Web-based survey aimed at CE providers was constructed
to elicit a description of the providers, users, and the activities offered.
This study revealed that participants had considerable interest in
distance education development. Since distance CE features are now

better known, this is a step toward the advancement and development of more and better distance programs as organizations can share their experiences and models for programs. Although research in continuing medical education demonstrates positive outcomes of online CE programs, the effectiveness of and learner satisfaction with interpersonal interaction in distance CE is lower (Sargeant, Curran, Jarvis-Selinger, Ferrier, Allen, Kirby, Ho, 2004). The results of this study demonstrate that, with integration of sound pedagogical instructional design, a need for distance-based CE could be met.

Interaction

Better programs would not be possible without the consideration of practitioner experiences that suggest that interacting with peers and mentors in the workplace provides the best environment for learning, which in turn enhances professional practice and professional judgment (Parboosingh, 2002). This assertion is supported by research findings that reaffirm two important principles in adult learning. First, we learn most naturally when faced with meaningful problem-solving experiences; second, learning results in action when constructed by the individual. This research supports the notion that, without sound pedagogical principles and theoretical considerations for interaction and learner experiences, quality distance CE will not be possible (Parboosingh, 2002).

Although the trend is to put more and more CE online, it has only been recently that pedagogical considerations for design and delivery are starting to be noted. For example, in recent years CE developers were looking at interactive strategies to enhance learning using activities such as "blogging" or reflective journaling. A study by Bouldin, Homes, and Fortenberry (2006) found that although reflective journaling can be used as a learner-centered assessment tool to determine whether students are actually making sense of the content discussed in class, the students described this activity as "busy work." This demonstrates the need for interaction to be an integral part of the course design, not just an added activity.

Davis (1999) reviewed randomized controlled trials on CE interventions and found personal interaction to be central to effective change in practice. Several studies reported that health care professionals seek confirmation and validation of current and new medical practices through their peers. Other studies confirmed the importance of interaction in changing professional behavior. However, researchers have not established which elements of the interactive process enable learning. This is despite the preference shown among physician groups that many prefer lectures, although this may include interaction if it is built into the design of the course.

Learning and practice cannot be separated when professionals work closely in specialty areas within the health care arena (Parboosingh, 2002). Interestingly however, physicians report that such interactions with colleagues are an important source of learning, and educators and course designers have only recently considered using the power of communities to foster learning through practice (Parboosingh, 2000). Membership within a learning community, however, has its responsibilities, because expectations and pressures from peers and mentors in a community of practice influenced standards for learning and practice. The significance of this finding tells us that continuing professional development providers should focus on meeting the learning needs of multidisciplinary communities of practice rather than individual learners. This research has implications for design considerations of CE courses.

More acceptable and effective methods for professional continuing education should be required to promote health care team member collaboration. It is thought that this collaboration would then encourage health care workers to interact with peers and mentors in order to frame issues, brainstorm, validate and share information, make decisions, and create management protocols, all of which contribute to learning in practice (Parboosingh, 2002). Physicians, however, were quick to note that if the CE was not directly related to their practice, then it would be a waste of their time.

QUALITY

As distance CE has grown steadily over the past several years, the quality has received limited attention in the medical literature, and few have attempted to establish or describe quality standards (Olson

& Shershneva, 2004). Standards can be used to synthesize practical knowledge, best practices, and research findings. They vary in their perspectives on quality, fall short of being comprehensive, and convey many elements that apply to distance CE. The conclusions are that published standards in the distance-education literature can provide valuable guidance to distance CE providers, and additional research is clearly needed into questions about what works in continuing education and why. The standards should be seen as instruments to achieve a higher goal while remaining cognizant of what it is that one is trying to achieve.

A framework for implementing technology-enabled knowledge translation into the health care culture was described by Ho, Block, Gondocz, Laprise, Perrier, Ryan, Thivierge, and Wenghofer (2004). They claim that this requires cultivation and acceptance in the domains of perceiving types of knowledge and ways in which clinicians acquire and apply knowledge in practice. Understanding the conceptual and contextual frameworks of information and communication technologies as applied to health care systems, comprehending essential issues in implementation of information, and communication technologies and strategies to take advantage of emerging opportunities, and finally, establishing a common and widely acceptable evaluation framework are all part of this translation as well. The successful transfer of knowledge from a technology-supported learning environment to practice, according to these authors, depends on a vision about the goals to be achieved, identification of cultural and political issues, human and financial resources, as well as legal, ethical, and technological limitations. This framework takes into account the complex considerations of CE design coupled with technical considerations and the ultimate purpose for delivery being that of practice change.

New developments in technology allow today's CE providers to meet more effectively the criteria necessary for effective continuing education (Harden, 2005). These include convenience, relevance, individualization, self-assessment, independent learning, and a systematic approach to learning. A case study conducted at the International Virtual Medical Schools in the United Kingdom (Harden, 2005) demonstrated how rapid growth of distance learning can alter undergraduate education and can have the potential to alter the nature of

CE. Key components include a bank of reusable learning objects, a virtual practice with virtual patients, a learning-outcomes framework, and self-assessment instruments. Learning is facilitated by a curriculum map, guided-learning resources, "ask the experts" opportunities, and collaboration or peer-to-peer learning. Researchers also found that distance learning provided a bridge between the cutting edge of education and training and outdated procedures embedded in institutions and professional organizations. It is often these organizations that can be credited for keeping health care professionals up to date with current practice issues.

If health care professionals are not kept up to date with current practice, the design and subsequently the quality of CE course offerings is only going to deteriorate. Without the keen attention and deliberate actions for incorporating research findings into new course design, the health care practitioners will ultimately not be achieving their goal of knowledge enhancement for the ultimate purpose of providing current, up-to-date patient care.

Strategies for Improving CE Offerings

Problem-solving strategies illustrate the contribution of theory to practice. The ability to frame and solve problems is central to the health care professional's level of competence. It is known that the ability to solve problems is tightly tied to one's knowledge in that area; therefore, problem solving ability varies markedly from case to case and from context to context. These findings have led to new understandings and revised theories about promoting the learning of problem solving. We now know that learners require a wide variety and number of opportunities and exemplars in learning how to solve problems so that they have many different problem-solving approaches from which to draw. Theory's iterative relationship with practice provides a powerful tool for improvement in the field.

Additional principles that should be applied to CE design should come from Chickering and Gamson's (1987) and Chickering and Ehrman's (1997) seminal works. These principles should be incorporated into the pedagogical design utilizing opportunities for active learning strategies, feedback, time on task and efficiency of delivery

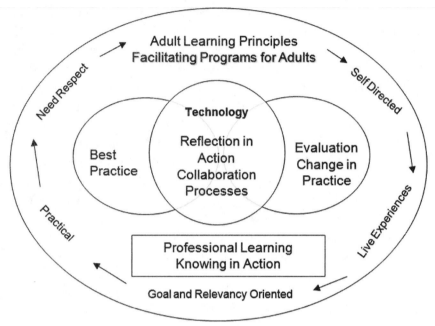

Figure 10.1 A model for CE design utilizing layered theory, best practices and evaluation.

utilizing technology, collaboration with peers, and interaction with faculty, setting high course expectations and showing respect for diversity. The model shown in Figure 10.1 depicts an approach for incorporating the multifaceted considerations necessary when designing quality CE. This model considers principles for adult learning, layered with considerations for the experiential learner, specifically in health care, in addition to the opportunity for social interaction, since this is known to support learning. This interaction could be technology supported, coupled with best practices for teaching with technology. Evaluation should also be built into the course design, because it is well documented that this area is often overlooked in CE relative to practice change.

The purpose of this chapter was to identify a multifaceted pedagogical approach for distance-based continuing education as evidenced by the distance-learning and the CE literature. This review also addressed current empirical studies on distance-based continuing education, which are also now starting to look at pedagogical design considerations by incorporating opportunities for interaction and principles from theoretical perspectives. Slotnick and Shersheva (2004) implied that several theoretical components can be applied in order to explain and support future design of technology-supported courses; however, this design must be cost efficient and effective. With the improvement in technology, computer and Web-based education have set the stage for dynamic, information-rich learning opportunities.

The importance of technology to health care professional development is growing rapidly and is echoed throughout the literature. Access to distance CE must be immediate, relevant, credible, easy to use, cost efficient, and effective. A sense of high utility demands content that is focused and well indexed in order to meet the health care professional's needs. The roles of the CE provider must be reshaped to include helping health care professionals seek and construct the kind of knowledge they need to improve patient care (Casebeer, et al., 2004).

In summary, distance-based CE currently lacks a theoretical underpinning, does not consider best practices for teaching, and does not utilize technology to enhance the quality of course offerings. Current research should apply what is known from the field of educational research coupled with what is known about the health professional as a learner in an attempt to deliver quality learning opportunities with better outcomes for practicing health care providers.

REFERENCES

Abrahamson, S., Baron, J., Elstein, A., Hammond, W., Holzman, G., Marlow, T., & Schulkin, J. (1999). Continuing medical education for life; eight principles. *Academic Medicine,* 74(12), 1288–1294.

Bouldin, A., Holmes, E., & Fortenberry, M., (2006). Blogging about course concepts: using technology for reflective journaling in a communications course. *American Journal of Pharmaceutical Education,* 70(4), 84.

Carriere, M., & Harvey, D. (2001). Current state of distance continuing medical education in North America. *Journal of Continuing Education in the Health Professions,* 21, 150–157.

Casebeer, L., Kristofco, R., Strasser, S., Reilly, M., Krishnamoorthy, P., Rabin, A., Zheng, S., Karp, S., & Myers, L. (2004). Standardizing evaluation of on-line continuing medical education: Physician knowledge, attitudes, and reflection on practice. *Journal of Continuing Education in the Health Professions,* 24, 68–75.

Chickering, A., & Ehrmann, S. (1996, October). Implementing the Seven Principles: Technology as lever, *AAHE Bulletin,* 3–6.

Chickering, A., & Gamson, Z. (1987, June). Seven principles for good practice in undergraduate education, *AAHE Bulletin.*

Cobb, S. (2004). Internet continuing education for health care professionals: An integrative review. *Journal of Continuing Education in the Health Professions,* 24, 171–180.

Curran, V. & Fleet, L. (2005). A review of evaluation outcomes of Web-based continuing medical education. *Medical Education,* 39(6), 561–567.

Davis, D., O'Brien, M., & Freemantle, N. (1999). Impact of formal continuing medical education: Do conferences, workshops, rounds, and other traditional continuing education activities change physician behavior or health care outcomes? *Journal of the American Medical Association,* 282, 867–874.

DeBourgh, G. (1999), Technology is the tool, teaching is the task: Student satisfaction in distance learning. Society for Information Technology & Teacher Education International Conference (10th, San Antonio, TX, February 28–March 4, 1999).

Dolcourt, J., Zuckerman, & Warner, K. (2006). Learners' decisions for attending pediatric grand rounds: A qualitative and quantitative study. *BMC Medical Education,* 6(26), 1–8.

Fox, R., (1991). New research agendas for CME: Organizing principles for the study of self-directed curricula for change. *Journal of Continuing Education in the Health Professions,* 11, 155–167.

Giguere, P., Formica, S., & Harding, W. (2004). Large-scale interaction strategies for Web-based professional development. *American Journal of Distance Education,* 18(4), 207–223.

Harden, R. (2005). A new vision for distance learning and continuing medical education. *Journal of Continuing Medical Education in the Health Professions,* 25, 45–51.

Heller, B., Oros, M., & Durney-Crowley, J. (2000). The future of nursing education: Ten trends to watch. *Nursing and Health Care Perspectives,* 21(1), 9–13.

Ho, K., Block, R., Gondocz, T., Laprise, P., Ryan, D., Thivierge, R., & Wenghofer, E. (2004). Technology-enabled knowledge translation; frameworks to promote research and practice. *Journal of Continuing Education in the Health Professions,* 24(2), 90–99.

Jung, I., Choi, C., Lim C., & Leem, J. (2004). Effects of different types of interaction on learning achievement, satisfaction, and participation in Web-based instruction. *Innovations in Education and Teaching International,* 39(2), 153–162.

Keane, D., Norman, G., & Vickers, J. (1991). The inadequacy of recent research on computer assisted instruction. *Academic Medicine,* 66, 444–448.

Knowles, M. (1970). *The modern practice of adult education: Andragogy versus pedagogy.* New York: The Association Press.

Moore, M., (1993). Transactional distance theory in D. Keegan (ed.). *Theoretical principles of distance education.* New York: Routledge.

Olson, C. & Shershneva, M. (2004). Setting quality standards for Web-based continuing medical education. *Journal of Continuing Education in the Health Professions,* 24, 100–111.

Parboosingh, J. (2002). Physician communities of practice: Where learning and practice are inseparable. *Journal of Continuing Education in the Health Professions,* 22, 230–236.

Sargeant, J., Curran, V., Jarvis-Selinger, S., Ferrier, S., Allen, M., Kirby, F., & Ho, K. (2004). Interactive on-line continuing medical education: Physicians' perceptions and experiences. *Journal of Continuing Education in the Health Professions,* 24, 227–236.

Shannon S. (2003). Adult learning and CME. *The Lancet,* 361(9353), 266–266s.

Sklar, B. (2006). Online CME: An update. Retrieved April 22, 2008, from http://www. cmelist.com/mastersthesis

Slotnick, M., Shershneva, M. (2004). Setting quality standards for Web based continuing medical education. *Journal of Continuing Education I in the Health Professions,* 24(2), 100–111.

Vygotsky, L. (1978). *Mind in Society: The development of higher psychological processes.* Cambridge, MA: Harvard University Press.

Zimitat, C. (2001). Designing effective on-line continuing medical education. *Medical Teacher,* (23)2, 117–122.

11 Using Technology in Teaching

CAROL A. O'NEIL

Using technology in teaching means including instructional media in learning environments for the purpose of communicating and enhancing content delivered to learners. Technology should allow for greater connectivity and greater collaboration, so both traditional and nontraditional students who have different technology needs will learn using technology (Campus Technology, n.d.). Jim Lengel (2008) outlines several uses and advantages for using technology in teaching:

- Productivity: technology allows students to be more productive and learn more in less time.
- Communication: technology enhances communication via e-mail between students and between teachers and students. Faculty office hours can be held in synchronous chat rooms in the course or through an instant messenger.
- Research: current information can be accessed through the Internet, thus allowing for current information in the classroom.

■ Media: teachers are using technologies and media to enhance their teaching.

■ Publishing: Teachers are using technology to compose slide shows, post Web sites, produce podcasts, and present and publish them to their students. Student assignments can include the same publishing activities (Lengel, 2008).

Technology does not ensure learning nor does it guarantee effective learning or teaching. Technology can facilitate basic skills and high-order critical thinking skills, and can provide a more creative and flexible teaching and learning process (Pennsylvania State, 2003–2007). Technology should be used because it is congruous with the learning objectives: the technology matches the learning objectives. For example, if an objective in a community health class is to describe the role of federal agencies in an emergency epidemic situation, the teacher could delineate observation points for the students to observe, and then show the movie *Outbreak*. The movie could be followed with a discussion of the observation points. Another example might be to ask students to conduct an Internet search to find and summarize prevalence and incidence data about chronic diseases in the United States. The learning objective might be to delineate sources of health-related data.

Here are some questions to consider when considering technology:

■ Is technology needed to achieve the learning goals and objectives?

■ Will the technology contribute to the learning process in a way that is not possible unless it is used?

■ Will the technology allow the students to engage in activities that they otherwise would not experience, such as a windshield survey in a high-crime community or a field trip to nursing museums?

■ Do students have access to the technology that you plan to use? (Pennsylvania State, 2003–2007).

The Horizon Report is an annual effort by the New Media Consortium (2008) to identify and describe emerging technologies.

Grassroots video and collaboration webs are currently used in education, yet they continue to emerge as popular technologies cited in this report. Grassroots video are such technologies as video clips from cell phones or minimal cost software. Collaboration webs are technologies that enable groups to engage in such activities as editing documents and holding meetings online. A third emerging technology is mobile devices, such as cell phones that can access the Internet and enable communication. A fourth emerging technology is the mashup, which combines different sources of information and communication into a single tool that will allow for a transformation in the way information is understood and represented. A fifth trend is toward collective intelligence in which information will be generated and shared by groups and communities; one example is Wikipedia. The next generation of emerging technologies includes social networking and social operating systems that will be organized around people rather than content. How well are you connected? Are you a connected academic? Take this quiz to find out: http://www.gotoquiz.com/the_connected_academic.

If you are feeling disconnected as a result of taking the connected academic quiz, this chapter will help you regain a feeling of connectedness by focusing on using technology as a method of delivery (hybrid or blended learning environments), a classroom teaching strategy (Course Response Systems and Course Presenter), an assessment or evaluation strategy (ePortfolios), and active learning strategies that can be used to supplement learning (wikis, social bookmarking, YouTube, podcasting).

METHOD OF DELIVERY

Technology can be used to structure a hybrid or blended learning environment. Hybrid or blended learning environments combine face-to-face learning with technology. Technology is not an add-on to the traditional course. The traditional course and the learning objectives should be evaluated to determine what learning objectives can be best met with technology. When part of the course is online, there is usually less face-to-face time. Osguthorpe and Graham (2003) cite three main reasons for using a hybrid or blended learning environment:

- Learning is more effective because it is more active and learner centered;
- Learning is more accessible, flexible, and interactive;
- Such learning environments are more cost effective.

An example of how face-to-face and technology can be integrated in hybrid learning environments is that the learning content is online and class time can be used for projects or group discussions. Faculty at Rensselaer Polytechnic Institute (McDaniel, 2007) redesigned a biology course so that the face-to-face lectures were replaced with Web-enhanced interactive modules. They compared the traditional model with the Web-enhanced strategies and found a significant increase in learning in the Web-enhanced course. Creedy (2007) examined Bachelor of Science in Nursing students' perception of a Web-enhanced learning environment. The Web-enhanced learning opportunities included online activities, quizzes, videos, and virtual laboratories in addition to on-campus and off-campus learning activities. Student satisfaction with the Web-enhanced program was associated with the level of technological skills and the perceived quality and usefulness of the Internet material. The authors conclude that students with good IT skills are more likely to perceive Web-enhanced material as useful. The advantage of using hybrid learning environments is that the best of traditional and technological strategies can be combined to design creative and flexible learning environments. The disadvantages are the faculty and student technological expertise and the availability of resources needed to combine class and technology experiences.

A question has been raised about class attendance and electronic course material. Billings-Gagliardi and Mazor (2007) studied first year medical students and surveyed them about their lecture-attendance decisions. They concluded that students made deliberate attendance decisions, and their decisions were influenced by previous experiences with the instructor, predictions about what would occur during class, their personal learning preferences, and learning needs at the time of the class. The authors conclude that increasing the availability of Web-enhanced material did not influence the students' decision to attend class.

CLASSROOM TEACHING STRATEGIES

Classroom Response Systems

Classroom Response Systems, also called CRS, audience response systems, and "clickers," are instructional technologies that actively involve the learner in the learning process through real-time engagement and discussion among students during class. Clickers need hardware (the clickers) and software (program needed to aggregate data from clickers). The cost is inexpensive, software is available online, and the clickers can be sold in the bookstore. Buff (n.d.) offers the following steps to use clickers in the classroom. Students purchase or obtain a clicker according to school policy. The teacher then poses a multiple-choice question displayed on a PowerPoint® slide in the classroom. Each student answers the question by using a handheld transmitter (called a clicker) that transmits an infrared or radio frequency signal to a receiver attached to the teacher's computer. The software on the teacher's computer aggregates the students' answers and displays the data that the students entered.

The most challenging step is to design clicker questions that will enhance the students' learning of the content. Bruff (n.d.) suggests asking the following types of questions:

- Factual Questions: Ask questions about key facts.
- Conceptual Questions: Ask questions focused on assessing an understanding of the principles.
- One-Best-Answer Questions: Include questions that have multiple answer choices.
- Opinion Questions: Include opinion questions that can engage students in discussions.
- Data Gathering Questions: Gather demographic, opinion, or other data from students.
- Questions Asking for Predictions: Ask questions that predict the outcome of a case study.

- Games: Use games to illustrate points about human behavior.
- Feedback on Teaching: Ask students for direct feedback on a class or activity.

Faculty can pose a question and ask for responses. This information provides faculty with an assessment of understanding of the material and with discussion material. If the students understand the material, the faculty can move to the next topic. If students do not understand the content, the faculty can ask students to consult with the person sitting next to them and respond a second time. Differences in answers can be discussed. Faculty can pose case studies or clinical problems and ask students for their opinions. Discussions can be based on the students' answers.

Preszler, et al. (2007) surveyed students in six biology classes about the impact of CRS on their learning experience. Students had favorable impressions of the use of response systems and thought the technology impacted their interest in the course, attendance, and understanding of course content. Lower division students were more positive about the experience than upper division students. The authors also studied the impact of clickers on exam grades and concluded that students in classrooms that used clickers scored higher on exams. Crossgrove and Curran (2008) also found that students were more satisfied and scored higher on exams in classes in which clickers were used. These authors found that the differences were more dramatic for nonbiology than biology majors in a biology course, and nonmajor students retained more information four months after the course ended.

Classroom Presenter

The University of Washington (n.d.) uses Classroom Presenter, a Tablet PC-based interaction system that allows for the real time integration of digital ink and electronic slides to send information back and forth between the teacher who is lecturing in the classroom and students in the classroom. It provides a mechanism for active learning in the classroom and creates mechanisms for feedback that support lecture presentation and classroom interaction.

Assessment or Evaluation Strategy

Electronic Portfolios (e-Portfolios)

E-Portfolios are electronic collections of accomplishments that exemplify growth. Designing an e-Portfolio is influenced by the need to function in a knowledge economy, the changing nature of learning, and the changing needs of the learner (Siemens, 2004). The e-Portfolio is a mechanism for expressing knowledge through means other than a transcript or a résumé. The portfolio can include artifacts that represent life experiences beyond the formal classroom, and the use of technology is familiar to the characteristics of today's learners (Siemens, 2004). The learner gathers the information and creates the collection. Universities can acquire the software and offer this option to students. The e-Portfolio is personal and learner centered. Information included in an e-Portfolio can include personal information, education, awards, coursework, faculty feedback, employment history, goals, personal values presentations, papers, workshops, and reflective comments (Siemens, 2004).

E-Portfolios are used at the Minnesota State Colleges and Universities, The Johns Hopkins University, and the University of North Carolina at Charlotte. EFolio Minnesota (n.d.) is a product of the Minnesota State Colleges and Universities in partnership with state workforce and education organizations. EFolio Minnesota is a multimedia electronic portfolio available to all citizens of Minnesota. Its focus is to create a living, personal showcase of education, career, and personal achievements.

The Johns Hopkins University Center for Technology in Education (n.d.) uses e-Portfolios for reflection, which they believe is critical to learning. The University of North Carolina at Charlotte College of Education (The University of North Carolina at Charlotte, n.d.) requires that education students design their e-Portfolio to satisfy the technology knowledge and application requirements necessary to be licensed to teach in North Carolina.

Universities can develop their own portfolio software, or they can use existing or commercial systems. The main implementation issues include obtaining the software and maintaining portfolios, providing security and privacy, and deciding on ownership and intellectual property rights of the portfolio (Lorenzo & Ittelson, 2005).

ACTIVE LEARNING STRATEGIES USING TECHNOLOGY

Podcasting

Podcasting is publishing course content to the Web. The most common uses are: as archives of classroom lectures, and supplementary class material, as content summaries and homework problems, and as student assignments, in which students can create a podcast in place of an oral presentation. There are three categories of activities involved in podcasting: file production, podcast publication, and delivery and playback (Deal, 2007). The most time-consuming activity is developing the podcast. This step requires planning and organizing the content and then recording the content. Hardware to record the content can be digital microphone or digital camera and software for editing the audio or video files. Technology support may be needed to publish the files to the Web. Students can subscribe, download, and listen to the podcast.

YouTube

YouTube is a video sharing Web site that allows users to post videos, watch videos, and post comments in a threaded discussion. To upload videos to YouTube, you must first create a free user account. To create videos, the author needs a Web cam and video maker (free downloads are available). Videos can be informational, entertaining, persuasive, and personal (EDUCAUSE, 2006). It has the power to engage, enlighten, and fascinate students and is used to supplement learning. The advantages of YouTube are that it is easy to use and free. It is a social networking tool that engages students, and allows for meeting new people, sharing opinions, and being part of a community (EDUCAUSE, 2006). YouTube can be used to find existing videos or create new videos (Durrant, n.d.).

Wiki

Wikis allow for easy, fast, and collaborative read-and-write Web sites to be built without the need for special software or a lot of training (CR 2.0, n.d.). It is easy and effective for collaboration and can be used in education for collaborative group projects (EDUCAUSE, 2005b). A wiki is a Web-publishing tool that can be used by a single individual, by multiple individuals who publish their own content to a single Web site, and by a fully collaborative community in which multiple individuals can work together on the same content (CR 2.0, n.d.). An example is Wikipedia, which allows anyone to edit any page.

Five elements are characteristic of wikis (CR 2.0, n.d.):

- The browser can be edited without the need for specialized programs;
- Links can be made to uncreated pages so organization can be created on-the-fly;
- The wikis are organized in chronological order, so even when changes are made the originals are retrievable;
- Discussion areas are available;
- Wiki's can be monitored so changes are communicated.

Students and teachers can create wiki Web pages that can be edited anytime and anywhere, thus allowing for group work and collaboration. Wikis can be used for: class notes, summaries, handouts, syllabi, course links, calendars, resources, and many others (CR 2.0, n.d.). Harris and Zeng (2008) used wikis in a health information management baccalaureate online course. Students were surveyed on the use of wikis for facilitating learning, student activities, reflective group interaction, and application to other courses. Data from 2006 and 2007 show that more than 50% of the students agree that wikis are effective for student activities. An average of 47% rated it an effective tool for facilitating learning, 44% agree it is a medium for reflective group interaction, and 37% suggest its application in other courses.

Social Bookmarking

Social bookmarking is a way to gather, organize, store, and share Internet sites. The sites are organized by tags that are designed by the author and can be accessed and shared with a group. The process starts with registering with a bookmarking site, choosing tags, and adding bookmarks to the site. The advantage for social bookmarking is the sharing and collaborating of resources about an area of interest. A disadvantage is that the author tags (EDUCAUSE, 2005a) are author driven and can be difficult for others to find. Social bookmarking is easy to use, and forming informal communities of interest is its main purpose (EDUCAUSE, 2005a). Social bookmarking allows for retrieving information, and students can use it to create directories of information and resources. It is more important to know how to retrieve information than to know information, and social bookmarking fulfills this purpose (EDUCAUSE, 2005a).

In summary, technology can enhance the learning environment. It must add to learning and be related to the learning objectives. Including technology allows for differing learning styles, active learning, and fun.

REFERENCES

Billings-Gagliardi, S. & Mazor, K. M. (2007). Student decisions about lecture attendance: Do electronic course materials matter? *Academic Medicine,* 82(10 Suppl), S73–76.

Bruff, D. (n.d.) Center for Teaching: Classroom Response Systems. Retrieved March 28, 2008, from http://www.vanderbilt.edu/cft/resources/teaching_resources/technology/crs.htm#questions

CR 2.0. (n.d.). Link to Classroom 2.0. Social network discussions: Wiki. Retrieved April 3, 2008, from http://www.classroom20wiki.com/Wikis

Campus Technology. (n.d.).Creating tomorrow's classrooms. Retrieved March 28, 2008, from http://campustechnology.com/mcv/resources/solutioncenters/center/wirelesstechnologies/article/?msid=1&id=40051&c1p=1

Creedy, D. K., Mitchell, M., Seaton-Sykes, P., Cooke, M., Patterson, E., Purcell, C., & Weeks, P. (2007). Evaluating a Web-enhanced bachelor of nursing curriculum: Perspectives of third-year students. *Journal of Nursing Education,* 46(10), 460–467.

Crossgrove, K., & Curran, K. L. (2008). Clickers in the large classroom: current research and best-practice tips. *CBE Life Science Education,* 7(1), 146–154.

Deal, A. (2007). Teaching with technology. White paper on podcasting. Retrieved March 29, 2008, from http://connect-cdn.educause.edu/files/CMU_Podcasting_Jun07.pdf

Durrand, E. (n.d.). How teachers can use video sharing for teaching: YouTube in education. Retrieved April 4, 2008, from http://www.metcomm.net/index.php?Itemid=120&id=109&option=com_content&task=view

EDUCAUSE. (2005a). 7 things you should know about social bookmarking. Retrieved April 5, 2008, from http://www.educause.edu/ir/library/pdf/ELI7001.pdf

EDUCAUSE. (2005b). 7 things you should know about wikis. Retrieved April 5, 2008, from http://www.educause.edu/ir/library/pdf/ELI7004.pdf

EDUCAUSE. (2006). 7 things you should know about YouTube. Retrieved April 5, 2008, from http://www.educause.edu/ir/library/pdf/ELI7018.pdf

eFolio Minnesota. (n.d.). Retrieved April 2, 2008, from http://www.efoliominnesota.com/index.asp?Type=NONE&SEC={116D5481-4358-483D-B413-309B7E654CD7}

Harris, S. T. & Zeng, X. (2008). Using wiki in an online record documentation systems course. *Perspectives in Health Information Management,* 5(1), 1–16.

The Johns Hopkins University Center for Technology in Education. (n.d.). The Johns Hopkins Digital Portfolio. Retrieved April 2, 2008, from http://olms.cte.jhu.edu/olms/output/page.php?id=2845

Lenger, J. (2008). Teachers, technology, and competence. Retrieved April 3, 2008, from http://www.powertolearn.com/articles/teaching_with_technology/article.shtml?ID=78

Lorenzo, G. & Ittloelson, J. (2005). An overview of e-portfolios. EDUCAUSE Learning Initiative. Retrieved April 3, 2008, from http://www.educause.edu/ir/library/pdf/ELI3001.pdf

McDaniel C. N., Lister, B. C., Hanna, M. H., & Roy, H. (2007). Increased learning observed in redesigned introductory biology course that employed Web-enhanced, interactive pedagogy. *CBE Live Science Education,* 6(3), 243–249.

New Media Consortium. (2008). The horizon report 2008 edition. Retrieved April 2, 2008, from http://www.educause.edu/ir/library/pdf/CSD5320.pdf

Osguthorpe, R. & Graham, R. (2003). Blended learning systems: Definitions and directions. *Quarterly Review of Distance Education,* 4(3), 227–234.

Pennsylvania State University. (2003–2007). Teaching and learning with technology. Retrieved April 3, 2008, from http://tlt.psu.edu/suggestions/research/media.shtml

Preszler, R. W., Dawe, A., Shuster, C. B., & Shuster, M. (2007). Assessment of the effects of student response systems on student learning and attitudes over a broad range of biology courses. *CBE Live Science Education,* 6(1), 29–41.

Siemens, G. (2004) EPortfolios. Elearning space. Retrieved April 2, 2008, from http://www.elearnspace.org/Articles/eportfolio.htm

University of North Carolina at Charlotte. (n.d.). College of Education ePortfolio. Retrieved April 3, 2008, from http://education.uncc.edu/ePortfolio/All_About.htm

University of Washington. (n.d.). UW classroom presenter. Retrieved April 2, 2008, from http://classroompresenter.cs.washington.edu

12 Educating Patients for Positive Behavior Change and Health Outcomes

BARBARA COVINGTON AND CAROL A. O'NEIL

Education in the health care field is benefiting tremendously from changes in both education and technology. No matter where education is needed, who specifically needs the education, or what number of learners the education will serve, more and more is becoming available. Challenges and new problems are still evolving with new technologies and the advances of the Internet and the World Wide Web. But in a time when access to care is benefiting from the changes in technology, technology and new media are breaking down barriers and opening up access to education that will allow for positive behavior changes and health outcomes.

This chapter covers education for consumers that is customized, individualized, and prescriptive. The differences between these three approaches to patient education are discussed, examples are offered, and research and theories underpinning the approaches are described. The steps to patient education include three phases: the assessment phase, the implementation phase, and the follow-up and evaluation phase, and each phase is described. In the assessment phase, educational needs are assessed. The educational prescription is developed, which includes customizing the four rights of education—the right information, right source, right dose, and right method of instruction. In the implementation phase, the role of the learner is emphasized, and the role of the practitioner is viewed as a facilitator of learning. The role and importance of follow-up and evaluation are explained. From the first step when the consumer either seeks out education or is directed to education by someone else, the importance of evaluation and the availability of tools to assist the provider and the consumer-patient are presented.

It is important first to understand the definition of patient education. Patient education is the "transfer of health-related knowledge from various health care sources to the patients themselves as well as the development of the necessary skills for integrating the knowledge into their lives" (Lewis, 2003, p. 88). Joint Commission on Accreditation of Health Care Organizations (2006) expands this definition to include that the knowledge gained will improve health. The commission outlines four purposes of patient education: disseminate knowledge, enhance coping, enhance self-care skills, and change behavior to maximize health.

Traditional sources of patient information for consumers have been pamphlets and other written material, videotapes and audiotapes, and multimedia. Information has been provided in print, on tapes, as recorded telephone messages, as videos or CDs and DVDs. Some sources of patient education material include hospitals, physician offices, health insurance companies, federal health sources (such as NIH), voluntary organizations (such as the American Heart Association) and commercial vendors. Patient education can be delivered through group programs or individual sessions, but for many years the focus has been the vendor, health agency, or provider identifying a need and investing the time and money into creating the educational resource. Most consumers learn about patient education materials, information, or classes from a healthcare encounter, direct mailing, school, or other informal source. Today, the consumer has new technologies and electronic communication sources that expand the world of education to real time, no matter where they are, what they are doing, or the time of day or night.

Computers have allowed patient education to broaden from individual and group education to education through the internet.

The advantages (Lewis, 2003) of computer-based patient education are that:

- Patients can seek out information at their convenience;
- Patients can access information via the Web;
- Web sources provide consistent information;
- Information can be tailored for the individual;
- Skills can be learned in controlled environments;
- Information can be used to support decisions.

Lewis (2003) reviewed the literature and concluded that patients who use the Web for education report:

- significant increases in knowledge through Web-based instruction;
- an improvement in self-care and self-management behaviors;
- stronger social support and perceived health;
- more confidence in decisions about health, increased adherence to treatment regimes, increased satisfaction and clinical outcomes.

Most of the information accessed via the Web relate to chronic disease, such as heart disease, arthritis, diabetes and oncology. The literature supports that patient information provided through traditional methods results in improved health. What evidence is there to support that teaching via computers or the Web is also effective? Wantland, et al. (2004) conducted a meta-analysis of changes in health behaviors between Web and non-Web patient education modalities. The findings showed an improvement in health outcomes in the Web group in knowledge gain and behavior change. In another study, an Interactive Multimedia Program for Asthma Control and Tracking was developed to study the outcomes of an asthma education program for children. Researchers concluded that using this program significantly increased asthma knowledge in children and caregivers. In addition, children experienced fewer asthma symptoms, made fewer visits to the emergency room and urgent visits to the physician, and used less medication than the control group (Krishna, et al., 2003). These findings are consistent with other studies reported in the literature. The Web has become a modality for disseminating information so much so, that there is an overabundance of health related information on the Web. But the warning is that with an overabundance of uncontrolled and unchecked health related information on the Web, some sites offer quality information, while others are lacking in quality.

Two examples of how the Web has been used to educate patients are seen in a preoperative teaching program and a dental anxiety support program. The first example of education using a computer and the Web is one used for preoperative teaching. Hering, et al. (2005) evaluated the use of a Web site as a method of disseminating supplemental information about preoperative teaching. Hering studied knowledge, satisfaction with anesthesia care, and anxiety. Two groups of preoperative patients were given information during their preoperative appointment. One group was offered the same information on the Web that could be accessed after the preoperative appointment. The results were that the group who accessed the information on the Web had a significant increase in knowledge and were more satisfied with their anesthesia care. The researchers found no differences in anxiety.

The second example expands into the dental field. The Web has been used to successfully provide information, advice, and support for dentally anxious and phobic patients who consider themselves to be isolated because of fear, stigma, or embarrassment (Buchanan & Coulson, 2007).

With all of the successes being referenced, it is important to remember that educating patients is a process comprising essential phases, and the most important phase is assessing the users. Stopp, et al. (2004) evaluated two computer-based information systems and found that they were underused, yet when they were used, the consumers were not satisfied. The designers in these two computer-based systems assumed what the consumers wanted and needed in building their systems. Thus a gap between the material and the needs of the consumer resulted. The authors conclude that the reason for the lack of success is that when designers create education systems, they need to be sensitive to the needs of the learners.

This focus on individualizing patient education is important for several reasons. One is that the reading level of information is high and not amenable to the reading levels of all consumers, so comprehension may be impacted (Graber, Roller, & Kaeble, 1999). The second is that consumers have access to a variety of sources for health information on the Web. Educators are concerned about the reliability of information and concerned about whether consumers who accessed the information were correctly interpreting the information (Wilson, 1999). The consumer must want to know about the topic, be ready to learn the information, and the information must be presented so it matches their learning style. Although Stopp, et al. (2004) was not successful in individualizing patient education through computer-based programs, a Web site to improve asthma care was successfully developed. An individualized approach for asthma patients was created so patients could develop questions for their health care provider before their appointment. The program included assessing the patient's knowledge and adherence to evidence-based clinical guidelines and providing individualized feedback based on the self-reported findings. Patients perceived the intervention as improving communication with their health care provider and improving their self care. Physicians rated the intervention as positive (Hartmann, et al., 2007).

McMullan (2006) reviewed the literature in search of how obtaining health information on the Internet (Web) affects the patient–health-professional relationship. She concludes that there is a shift in participation of the patient from a passive to an active role in seeking health information. Health professionals are responding in three ways: assuming a health-professional-centered relationship in which the professional is the expert; engaging in a patient-centered relationship, which focuses on collaboratively accessing information; and the Internet prescription approach, in which the health professional guides patients to reliable health information.

Brooks (2001) suggests that the nurse has a high level of interaction with the patient, family, and health care team and is the appropriate healthcare provider to conduct an initial assessment of learning need and then to develop a prescribed educational plan that will teach and reinforce learning. The skills the nurse needs to individualize and prescribe learning are to be able to evaluate and critique Web sites and patient education material and to be able to match the material to the consumer's literacy level, learning style, and information needed.

Consumers need to be warned that all information on the Web is not reliable information. Consumers need to be taught to assess the information on the Web through the three Cs: content, commerce, and connectivity of the information. The Health On the Net Foundation (n.d.) describes reliable information as showing evidence that the content is valid, that there is clear disclosure if the Web site is commercially supported, and the connectivity needs of the information to the needs of the consumer. Brooks (2001) suggested a fourth C: communication. Communication is assessing the patient's learning needs and the information that is available on the Web and individualizing and prescribing learning to meet learning needs. The health care provider is a key player in this communication. But there is a question about the role of the health care provider and the cost-benefit relationship of Web-based patient education (Lewis, 2003).

The Patient Education Institute Web site (www.patient-education. com) shares a definition for education prescription or patient education as a solution: the health care provider asks the patient to do something and the patients does it. With the number of national disease-specific organizations, medical organizations, and federal health-related agencies joining the movement to provide an individualized education prescription approach, quality resources on the Web are now more available to the patient, her family, and her associates, with or without health care provider interventions. It has become even more important for the healthcare providers, including nurses, to educate their patients on the steps they need to take to help insure that they are getting correct and reliable information.

ASSESSING EDUCATIONAL LEARNING NEEDS

Assessing learning needs is the key to successful learning outcomes. In addition to the content, providing targeted and appropriate patient education can be accomplished by considering the patient's values, literacy, culture, folk beliefs, alternative medical practices, spirituality, country of origin, educational level, and socioeconomic status (JCAHO, 2006). The needs of a group or needs of the individual can be assessed. JCAHO (2006) suggests guidelines for assessing the needs of a group. In determining the needs of groups, data can be collected by observation, questionnaires, interviews, group discussions and focus groups, tests, and secondary data analysis. Further, the individual characteristics of the patient and family that need to be considered are age, culture, patient goals and preferences, learning style, and readiness to learn (JCAHO, 2006).

The number of hospitals, universities, and health specialty organizations that include consumer and patient education on the Web continues to increase weekly. Individualized prescriptive educational plans can be created by the health care provider or the patient-consumer can create his own after he conducts his own self-assessment of learning needs. Regardless of approach, the assessment of learning needs should be objective. Checklists and help sheets are available online, in the literature, and in texts. Several are included at the end of this chapter. Some examples include:

- Better Diabetes Care by the National Institute of Health can be found at the National Diabetes Education Program Web site;
- Educational needs assessments of adult chronic hepatitis type C patients undergoing antiviral therapy can be found at Columbia University Libraries or Mayo Clinic's Health Oasis with its medical and health information and tools for patients or consumers
- Children's Hospital Medical Center of Cincinnati provides patient education information on pediatric diseases, procedure, treatments.

Now virtual hospitals are being built on the Web and are providing one-stop health education, which is often prescriptive or tailored by the consumer or patient to meet her own needs. Med Help International is one such virtual medical center for patients. This Web site provides patient information along with medical and health advice. In fact, interactive question and answer discussions forums are actually staffed by doctors from leading medical centers. Following the assessment, the educational prescription can be written by the provider or the patient/consumer. The patient/consumer is given the prescriptive plan, but this does not guarantee that it will be followed. The best way to ensure that the plan will be followed is to involve the patient-consumer in the planning process.

The patient or consumer must play an active role in participating in the assessment phase, but this does not mean that the care provider is out of the process. One approach is to prescreen selected Web sites or educational materials. The provider then completes the assessment with the patient and writes the educational prescription for the patient. The patient is then directed to the location of the educational material or provided with the material. The care provider may choose to set up computers in the waiting room or in a private area or set up educational materials to run on kiosks or multimedia viewing units. Doctors in Akron, Ohio, provide patient education prescriptions that include the disease or condition name and a list of seven Web sites where the patient and his family can learn about the condition or disease (Akron Beacon Journal, 2007).

On the other end of the spectrum, health care providers can write the educational prescription to access Web-based repositories filled with quality information and tutorials or other reusable learning objects. The information can be accessed and assembled to meet individual patient educational needs. One such site is described by Luke, Atack, Chien, MacDonald, Neligan, Wiljer, & Winter (2006). Their interdisciplinary health care team project is focused on Patient Education Prescriptions that are related to chronic diseases. They evaluated the information on the Web for clinical relevance to the patient and tailored it to maximize the effectiveness of the materials for the individual patient. The online patient education material is placed in a clinical learning object Web-based repository for access.

The customization of the patient prescription, at a minimum, needs to include the correct information to meet the learning need; the right source for the information; the correct dose or amount of information, including the number of times or other measures to indicate how often the patient should review the information or practice the skill; the right method of instruction for the patient; and information that is evidence based.

IMPLEMENTATION OF THE PRESCRIPTION

Once the information is customized, it is implemented. Again the patient-consumer is assuming responsibility for this step. Health care providers may be facilitators or coaches in this step, but ultimately the patient is in the lead. The individualized approach in patient education is not just successful for the adult population; children, adolescents, and elderly report success as well. Since a return on investment is often a concern in developing Web sites or repositories for the educational materials, the customization can be constructed so that greatest number of patient-consumers have access to the material, complete individual assessments, and implement their own prescription. In one Internet-based intervention for youth called Food, Fun, and Fitness Internet Program for Girls, Thompson (2008) found that an eight-week Internet-based obesity prevention program could be successful both for participation and individual successes.

FOLLOW-UP AND EVALUATION OF THE PRESCRIPTION

The final two steps in this process are follow-up and evaluation. By building in both of these when the patient-consumer's individualized education prescription is created, the learner continues to feel connected and not isolated. The follow-up step may take place in person, on phone, by e-mail, on a discussion board, or some combination of these. This step can be completed in one meeting or over a period of time. The follow-up must be appropriately timed for the learner's unique characteristics and for the tasks that are to be accomplished in the educational prescription. For example, if the prescription includes the objective that the client will report the signs and symptoms to the health care provider, the follow-up might need to be within a day or two and may be through a telephone call or e-mail. If it states that the client will verbalize an understanding of ways to maintain a specific infusion rate when wearing an implanted insulin device, the prescription might include online education about the device and its maintenance and include multimedia presentations. Follow-up might be based on the patient's need. The strength of this approach is that the care provider does not have the sole responsibility to follow up with each patient, and the patient herself can participate in selecting the method of follow-up. The educational process is a partnership with the provider becoming the resource or guide and the patient continuing in the role of assuming responsibility for self-management of the process. While they maintain the lead role in completing the prescription, the provider's follow-up allows reassessment of progress and support that can be further modified as needed over time.

In the final step of evaluation, the success of this step comes from the first and second steps. The more thorough the assessment and the more appropriate and individualized the prescription, the easier it will be to evaluate outcomes. Numerous Web sites, books, and articles are available for creating evaluation tools. The evaluation should consider a number of perspectives. The evaluation should include success in terms of the four Cs mentioned earlier in this chapter and in terms of the relationship of the outcomes to the patient's health care and educational objectives. For example, the prescriptive health education program included a new diabetic adult learning how to administer insulin following an initial one-to-one teaching session, review of tutorials, and participation in the clinic's online forum for new diabetics.

The evaluation for success would need to include patient feedback on her success in assuming responsibility for her disease management, including her skills and knowledge gain from the Web tutorials. Fortunately, patient educators do not have to create all the evaluation tools. The National Institute of Health provides examples of evaluations for patient learning programs. One example is from the National Heart Lung Book Institute Web site. This Web site includes the full programs and online options with standards and evidence-based practice supporting information. The Web site is listed at the end of the chapter in the resource list.

On a more state or local level, resources are often located at university Web sites or state initiatives to improve the health education of their citizens. These programs and Web sites often target national health concerns and or specific chronic diseases and health issues for that state. They are usually not fully individualized in a prescriptive nature but are customized to the state's population in regards the unique demographics of the citizens, their languages and cultures, and to the four rights of education (right information, right source, right dose, and right method of instruction), in addition to being evidence based. These sites are often like visiting a shopping mall. The visitor can look at the Web site home page as a directory and select which path to take based on her role (healthcare provider, consumer, child, or adult) or by their purpose (consumer education, constructing educational programs, or intervention). One university Web site is the University of California Davis Health System. Within their continuing nursing education Web site, there is patient educational material and a check list.

In summary, this chapter focused on patient education as the transfer of knowledge for the purpose of integrating this knowledge to change health outcomes. By using evidence-based approaches to education for the patient and by knowing how to seek out or create quality sources for educational materials, patient-consumers and health providers can create customized, individualized, and prescriptive health education plans. Implementing, follow-up and evaluating the health education plans will lead to positive behavior change and positive health outcomes.

ONLINE RESOURCES FOR PATIENT AND FAMILY EDUCATION

Children's Hospital Medical Center of Cincinnati: Cincinnati Ohio Children's Hospital provides patient education information about pediatric diseases, procedures, treatments and more. http://www.cincinnatichildrens.org/health/info

Enhancement, Inc: Enhancement, Inc. is a nonprofit foundation whose purpose is to teach and disseminate material relating to health and wellness. Site includes information about breast cancer. http://www.enhancementinc.com

Health Promotion and Disease Prevention: Healthful Life Project is for all adults to promote longer and healthier lives through health promotion and disease prevention activities. University of Medicine and Dentistry of New Jersey and Roche. http://healthfullife.umdnj.edu

Healthfinder: Healthfinder® is a free guide to reliable health information, sponsored by the U.S. Department of Health and Human Services. http://www.healthfinder.gov

Amarillo Medical Specialist LLP: Uses patient portals to allow patients access to their laboratory results, to make appointments, review medications and ask questions. Health information is provided. http://www.amarillomed.com/index.htm

JAMA'S Patient Education Pages: The full text of patient education articles from the *Journal of the American Medical Association.* http://jama.ama-assn.org/cgi/collection/patient_page

Lab Tests Online: Lab Tests Online offers patient education to help health care consumers better manage their care. A public resource on clinical lab testing from the professionals who do the testing. Peer reviewed, noncommercial, public site. http://www.labtestsonline.org

Mayo Clinic Health Oasis: Mayo Clinic offers award-winning medical and health information and tools for healthy living. http://www.mayoclinic.com/index.cfm

Med Help International: The Virtual Medical Center for Patients provides patient information, medical, and health advice. The site includes interactive question and answer forums staffed by online doctors from leading medical centers. There is an extensive library of articles on all diseases and health conditions, specializing in areas such as heart disease, neurology, child behavior, etc. http://www.medhelp.org

Medifocus Patient Research Guides: Home to over 120 complete medical guides and treatment options on diseases and other medical conditions. Guides available for purchase. http://www.medifocus.com

National Council on Patient Information and Education (NCPIE): This site is designed to help consumers make sound decisions about the use of medicines, and to stimulate and improve communication between consumers and health care professionals. National Council for Patient Information and Education. http://www.talkaboutrx.org

Netwellness.org: Experts in wellness, health, medicine, diet, drugs, and fitness offer information on over 100 topics. University of Cincinnati, The Ohio State University, and Case Western University. http://www.netwellness.org

NOAH: Health Topics and Resources: New York Online Access to Health is a metasite of listings by topic and source with the added bonus of offering a large selection of health information materials in Spanish as well as English. http://www.noah-health.org/en/search/health.html

Ohio State University's Patient Education Documents: The Ohio State University Medical Center Patient Education Materials covers an extensive list of medical and surgical conditions. Documents are available in .pdf format. http://medicalcenter.osu.edu/patientcare/patient_education/?CFID=14515359&CFTOKEN=59064758

Why Doctors Order Laboratory Tests: Nemours Foundation. This site provides parents with important facts about common lab tests, from bone scans to ultrasounds. http://www.kidshealth.org/parent/system/medical/labtest2.html

REFERENCES

Akron Beacon Journal. (2007). Retrieved on April 22, 2008, from www.healthleadersmedia.com/content_redirect.cfm?content_id=88840

Brooks, B. A. (2001). Using the Internet for patient education. *Orthopaedic Nursing, 20*(5), 69–77.

Buchanan, H. & Coulson, N. S. (2007). Accessing dental anxiety online support groups: An exploratory qualitative study of motives and experiences. *Patient Education and Counseling, 66,* 263–269.

Graber, M. A., Roller, C. M., & Kaeble, B. (1999). Readability levels of patient education material on the World Wide Web. *Journal of Family Practice, 48*(1), 58–61.

Hartmann C. W. et al. (2007). A Web site to improve asthma care by suggesting patient questions for physicians: Qualitative analysis of use. *Journal of Medical Internet Research*, 9(1).

Health On the Net Foundation. (n.d.) Retrieved on April 26, 2008, from http://www.hon.ch

Hering, K., Harvan, J., D'Angelo, M., & Jasinski, D. (2005). The use of a computer Web site prior to scheduled surgery (a pilot study): Impact on patient information, acquisition, anxiety level, and overall satisfaction with anesthesia care. *American Association of Nurse Anesthetists Journal*, 73(1), 29–33.

Joint Commission on Accreditation of Health Care Organizations (2006). *The Joint Commission Guide to Patient and Family Education*.

Krishna, S., et al. (2003). Internet-enabled interactive multimedia asthma education program: A randomized trial. *Pediatrics*, 111(3), 503–510.

Lewis, D. (2003). Computers in patient education. *CIN: Computers, Informatics, Nursing*, 21(2), 88–96.

Luke, R., Atack, L., Chien, E., MacDonald, S., Neligan, D., Wiljer, D., & Winter, T. (2006). Giving patients a PEPTalk: The patient education prescription project. T-space University of Toronto. Retrieved April 22, 2008, from http://tspacetest.library.utoronto.ca:8080/handle/1778/23900

McMullan, M. (2006). Patients using the Internet to obtain health information: How this affects the patient-health professional relationship. *Patient Education and Counseling*, 63, 24–28.

Thompson, D., Varanowski, K., Watson, K., Canada, A., Bhatt, R., Liu, Y., & Zakeri, I. (2008). Food, Fun and Fitness: Internet program for girls: influencing log-on rate. *Health Education Research*, 23(2), 228–237.

Wantland, D. J. (2004). The effectiveness of Web-based vs. non-Web-based interventions: A meta-analysis. *Journal of Medical Internet Research*, 6(4).

Wilson, S. M. (1999). Impact of the Internet on primary care staff in Glasgow. *Journal of Medical Internet Research*, 19(2), 7.

Index

A

Academic integrity, and student identification, 119
Accessibility
  and learner preferences, 157–158
  of technology, 124–125
Accreditation, 55
Active learning
  cognitive apprenticeship, 79–80, 109
  constructivism and, 27–28
  problem-based learning, 107–109
  Web quest resources, 106–107
Administrative support, for online learners, 40
Admissions process, 44
Adult learners
  continuing education for, 155–156
  student characteristics, 21–22
Advising guidelines, 40–42, 44–45
Agenda, for courses, 119–120
Amarillo Medial Specialist LLP, 189
American Association of Colleges of Nursing
  distance education, white paper on, 13, 67–71
  institutional strategic plans, 36–37
American Distance Education Consortium, strategic plan, 37–38
Americans with Disabilities Act, 124–125
Assessment. *See also* Evaluation
  criterion-referenced assessment, 136
  definition, 141
  electronic portfolios (e-portfolios) in, 173
  elements of, 139
  grading (*see* Grading)
  initial, 142–143
  instructional design considerations, 95–96
  in laboratory courses, 80–81
  of learning styles, 22–25
  methods, 144–145
  Model for Assessing and Evaluating Learning Online, 140–142
  of patient learning needs, 184–186
  student self-assessment, 43–44, 62–63, 126–128
  traditional, 136
  types of, 140
Association of College and Research Libraries, service guidelines, 47–49
Asthma education program, 181–182, 183
Asynchronous interaction
  definition, 2
  overview, 101–104
  types of, 92–93
Asynchronous Learning Networks, course design process, 95
Audience response systems. *See* Classroom Response Systems
Automation, 7

B

Behaviorism, 26–27. *See also* Guided constructivism
Best practices
  for online environments, 5–7
  in student support services, 42–43
Biography, as community building tool, 105–106
Blackboard (course management system), 58
Blended learning (hybrid courses)
  definition, 1–2
  reconceptualizing learning material, 74–75
  technology for, 169–171
Bodily-kinesthetic intelligence, 23

C

Campus Computing, 8–9
Chat meetings, 104
Children's Hospital Medical Center,
        Cincinnati, 185, 189
Class attendance, 170
Classroom Presenter, 172
Classroom Response Systems, 171–172
Clickers, 171–172
Clinical courses, 81–82
Cognition, 139
Cognitive apprenticeship, 79–80, 109
Collaboration
    course management, role in, 114–115
    inter-institutional (*see individual
        organizations*)
    learning teams, 103–104
    peer review (*see* Peer review)
Collaboration webs, 169
Communication
    asynchronous, 101–104
    synchronous, 104–105
Community building, 105–109
Computer use, statistics on, 8–10
Connecticut Distance Learning
        Consortium, 39
Consortia. *See individual organizations*
Constructivism
    and evaluation, 136–139
    in instructional design, 84–85
    overview, 27–29
Consumer health informatics, 10. *See
        also* Patient education
Continuing education
    for adult learners, 155–156
    distance-based (*see* Distance-based
        continuing education)
    instructional material design, 161–162
    model for CE Design, 162
    and pedagogy, 154–155
    social interaction and, 156–157
Continuing medical education, 12–13
Copyright law
    exclusive rights, limitations on, 54–56
    faculty training on, 51–52
Counseling services, 40
Course management
    agenda, 119–120
    collaboration, 114–115
    grading, 118–119, 145
    schedule, 117–118

syllabus, use of, 116–117, 129–133
Course management systems
    comparison of, 60–62
    faculty training in, 63–64
    overview, 57–59
    software, 47, 58, 60, 62
    for students, 62–63
Courses
    adaptation for online learning (*see*
        Reconceptualization, of learning
        material)
    design of (*see* Instructional design)
    types (*see* Clinical courses; Laboratory
        courses)
Course schedule, 117–118
Criterion-referenced assessment, 136

D

Dental anxiety support program, 182
Department of Education, Learning
        Anytime Anywhere Partnership, 8
Designing online environments
    course organization, 88
    design model, 94–96
    interacting, 92–93
    navigation, 91
    page layout, 92
    purpose, 87
    target population, 85
Discussion questions
    design of, 115–116
    as socialization tool, 86
Distance-based continuing education
    current issues, 152–154
    interaction, role of, 158–159
    pedagogical considerations, 157
    quality of, 159–163
    Web-based, 12–13
Distance education
    American Association of Colleges of
        Nursing white paper, 13, 67–71
    continuing education (*see* Distance-
        based continuing education)
    definition, 1
    historical perspective, 2–8
    infrastructure guidelines, 36
    Innovations in Distance Education
        project, 87
    for nursing students, 13–15
Diversity issues, 123–125
Duke University, clinical experiences, 81

E

Educational theories
  behavioral theory, 26–27
  constructivist theory, 27–29
  in online learning environment design,
    31–32
  social interaction, 29–30
EduTools, delivery system comparison,
    60, 61
Efolio Minnesota, 173
Electronic portfolios (e-portfolios), 144,
    173
Enhancement, Inc., 189
E-Pack, 62
eTutoring programs, 39
Evaluation. *See also* Assessment
  definition, 135
  Model for Assessing and Evaluating
    Learning Online, 140–142
  of patient education prescriptions,
    187–189
  peer review in, 146
  precourse, 145
  purposes of, 140
  types of, 141 (*see also individual
    types*)
Examinations
  as assessment tool, 144
  question types (*see* Discussion
    questions)
  student identification methods, 119
Existential intelligence, 24

F

Face to face learning, 18
Faculty
  asynchronous interaction with
    students, 101–102
  competencies, 63–64
  reconceptualizing learning material,
    70
  role of, 112–113
  training of, 49–52, 63–64
Faculty workload, definition, 50–51
Fair use, of copyrighted material, 56. *See
    also* Copyright law
Feedback
  characteristics of, 121–122
  continuous, 143–144
  importance of, 120–121
Financial aid, 46

Formative evaluation
  definition, 141
  techniques, 147

G

GIGO rule, 18
Grading. *See also* Assessment
  information for students, 118–119
  rubrics, 145
Graduate studies, in nursing, 17–18
Group collaboration, 103–104
Guided constructivism, 84–87

H

Healthfinder, 189
Health informatics, 10. *See also* Patient
    education
Health On the Net Foundation,
    information reliability guidelines,
    184
Health Promotion and Disease
    Prevention, 189
The Horizon Report, 9, 168
Hybrid courses. *See* Blended learning
    (hybrid courses)

I

Identification methods, 119
Illinois Online Network
  elements of online programs, 19–20
  faculty role, 112–113
  student self-evaluation, 126–128
  successful students, characteristics of,
    32–33
Index of Learning Style, 23
Indiana Higher Education
    Telecommunication System
  copyright law compliance, 51–52
  faculty development principles, 49–50
Infrastructure
  information technology, 38–40
  institutional considerations, 36–38
  library services, 47–49
  student support services, 40–43
Innovations in Distance Education
    project
  learning goals, 87
  multimedia use, 90–91
Institutional considerations
  collaborations, inter-institutional,
    39–40

course management system selection, 59
identification of students, 119
infrastructure, 36–38
in reconceptualizing learning material, 68–69
Instructional design
components of, 83–84
for continuing education programs, 161–162
course objectives, 87
course organization, 88–94
discussion questions, 115–116
student characteristics and, 126
target population and, 85–87
techniques, 95–96
Instructional media
Blackboard (course management system), 58
Classroom Response Systems, 171–172
live chat meetings, 104
mashup (emerging technology), 169
Moodle (course management system), 58
streaming media (Live-Live, Webcasting), 60, 62
television, 3
videoconferencing, 82, 104–105
Web quests, 106–107
Wiki, 174–175
YouTube, 174
Intellectual property, 51–52
Intelligence, types of, 23–24, 25
Interaction
asynchronous communication, 2, 92, 93, 101–104
in distance-based continuing education, 158–159
importance of, 99–101
instructional design considerations for, 92–94
interpersonal intelligence, 23, 25
intrapersonal intelligence, 24, 25
social interaction, 156–157
synchronous communication, 2, 104–105
Internet etiquette, 122
Interpersonal intelligence, 23, 25
Intrapersonal intelligence, 24, 25
Iowa Communications Network, 39–40

J
Johns Hopkins University Center for Technology in Education, e-Portfolio use, 173
Journal of the American Medical Association, patient education resources, 189

K
Knowles, Malcolm, 21

L
Laboratory courses, 79–80
Lab Tests Online, 190
Learner preferences, 157–158
Learning
cognitive apprenticeship, 79–80, 109
constructivism and, 27–28
goals, guiding principles for, 87
outcomes, traditional versus distance technology, 4
problem-based learning, 107–109
styles, 22–25
Web quest resources, 106–107
Learning Anytime Anywhere Partnership, 8
Learning teams, 103–104
Legal considerations. *See* Copyright law
Library services, 47–49
Live chat meetings, 104
Live-Live. *See* Streaming media
Logical-mathematical intelligence, 23, 25
Logs, student maintained, 82. *See also* Reflective journaling

M
Mashup (emerging technology), 169
Mathematical-logical intelligence, 23, 25
Mayo Clinic, Health Oasis, 185, 190
Med Health International, 185–186, 190
Mediated instructional activities, 55
Medifocus Patient Research Guides, 190
Mental models
for gerontological nursing course, 88–89
overview, 75–78
Metcalf's Law, 10

Model for Assessing and Evaluating Learning Online, 140–142
Moodle (course management system), 58
Moore's Law, 10
Multimedia use, 90–91
Multiple Intelligences theory, 23–24, 25
Musical-rhythmical intelligence, 23, 25
Myers-Briggs Type Indicator, 24

N
National Academic Advising Association Technology in Advising Commission
advising standards, 44–45
student support services policy, 40–42
National Council on Patient Information and Education, 190
National Diabetes Education Program, 185
National Education Association, effective education criteria, 20
National Institute of Health, patient learning program evaluation, 185, 188
Naturalist intelligence, 24, 25
Nemours Foundation, 190
Netiquette, 122
Netwellness.org, 190
New York Online Access to Health (NOAH), 190
Norm-referenced assessment, 136
No significant difference phenomenon, 4
Nurses
patient education, role in, 183–184, 186
professional association (*see* American Association of Colleges of Nursing)
Nursing education
certification examination review courses, 12–13
computer competencies, 63
continuing education (*see* Continuing education)
delivery systems (*see* Course management systems)
distance education, 13–15
educational theories and course design, 31–32
graduate studies in, 17–18
infrastructure considerations, 36–37

internet use and curriculum change, 11
gerontological nursing course, 88–89
online courses, decision to offer (*see* Reconceptualization, of learning material)
socialization among students, 86
Web quests for, 106–107

O
Ohio State University, patient education resources, 190
Online learning environment
course characteristics, 19–20
course design (*see* Reconceptualization, of learning material)
definition, 2
delivery systems (*see* Course management systems)
educational theories and design of, 31–32
infrastructure (*see* Infrastructure)
Model for Assessing and Evaluating Learning Online, 140–142
overview, 1–2
versus traditional learning, 18–19
Online universities, for graduate studies, 17–18
Open-source system, 58

P
Patient education
computer-based, 180–182
consumer health informatics, 10
definition, 180
education prescription, 184
follow-up phase, 187–189
implementation phase, 187
individualized, 182–183, 186
learning needs, 184–186
nursing curricula changes, 11
online resources, 189–190
phases in, 179–180
professional relationships in, 183–184
reliability, of information, 184
Patient Education Institute, 184
Pavlov, Ivan, 26
Pedagogy
and continuing education, 154–155
of online learning, 20–21
and reconceptualizing learning material, 78–79

Peer review
  criteria, 146
  process, 137–138
Pennsylvania State University
  distance education guidelines, 36
  faculty development course, 50
Personal readiness assessment, 43–44
Podcasting, 174
Portfolios (e-portfolios), 144, 173
Precourse evaluation, 141, 145–146
Preoperative patient teaching program,
    182
Principles of Good Practice, 5–7
Problem-based learning, 107–109
Professional associations. *See individual
    associations*
Professional relationships, in patient
    education, 183–184

Q
QuestionMark, 62

R
Reconceptualization, of learning
    material
  blended learning, 74–75
  clinical courses, 81–82
  decision making process, 67–74
  example, 76–78
  laboratory courses, 79–80
  mental models, use of, 75–78
  pedagogy, 78–79
Reflective journaling, 158. *See also* Logs,
    student maintained
Registration of students, 46–47
Resources for patient and family
    education, 189
Rubrics, 145

S
Sequence, of course, 120
Skinner, B. F., 26
Social bookmarking, 175–176
Social interaction, 29–30
  and continuing education, 156
Software
  course management systems,
      enhancements to, 60, 62
  for identification, 119
  portfolios, 173
  for student registration, 47

Stimulus-response studies, 26–27
Streaming media (Live-Live,
      Webcasting), 60, 62
Students
  adult learners, 21–22, 155–156
  asynchronous interaction, with other
      students, 101–102
  characteristics of, 21–22, 32–33
  expectations of, 128–129
  initial assessment of, 142–143
  prospective, support for, 43–46
  in reconceptualizing learning
      material, 71
  role, 125–128
  self-assessment, 44, 62–63, 126–128
  technology needs of, 62–63
Student support services
  availability, 40–42
  best practices, 42–43
  for prospective students, 43–46
Successive approximations process, 27
Summative evaluation
  definition, 141
  in formative evaluation, 147
Syllabus
  as course management tool, 116–119
  sample, 129–133
Synchronous interaction, 2, 92–93,
      104–105

T
Technology
  accessibility of, 124–125
  for active learning strategies,
      174–176
  advantages of, 167–168
  for blended learning, 169–171
  for classroom strategies, 171–173
  collaboration, inter-institutional, 39–40
  course management systems (*see*
      Course management systems)
  emerging tools, 169
  infrastructure (*see* Infrastructure)
  learning, role in, 30–31
  multimedia use, 90–91
  nursing education, role in, 13–14
  in reconceptualizing learning
      material, 70
  requirements, 38–39
  streaming media, 60, 62
  student requirements, 62–63

Television, as instructional medium, 3
Textbooks, 116–117
Thorndike, Edward, 26
Time commitment of students, 127
Traditional learning
versus constructivism, 27–28
versus online, 18–19

U
University of Arizona, graduate nursing program, 18
University of California, Instructional Enhancement Initiative, 7–8
University of Maryland
elements of learning online, 20
graduate nursing programs, 18
student assessment tools, 63

V
VARK (assessment method), 23
Verbal-linguistic intelligence, 23, 25
Videoconferencing, 82
synchronous, 104–105
Visual-spatial intelligence, 23, 25

W
Watson, John B., 26
Web-based patient education, 180–184
Webcasting. *See* Streaming media
Web Initiative in Teaching Project
formative evaluation questions, 147
peer review process, 146, 148
Web quests, 106–107
Western Cooperative for Telecommunications Education, student support service guidelines, 45–46
Western Interstate Commission for Higher Education
resource sharing, 39
student support service guidelines, 42–43
Why Doctors Order Laboratory Tests, 190
Wiki, 174–175

Y
YouTube, 174

Z
Zone of proximal development, 29, 156

SPRINGER PUBLISHING COMPANY

Nursing Leadership

A Concise Encyclopedia

Editor-in-Chief:

Harriet R. Feldman, PhD, RN, FAAN

Associate Editors:

Marilyn Jaffe-Ruiz, EdD, RN
Margaret L. McClure, RN, EdD, FAAN
Martha J. Greenberg, PhD, RN
Thomas D. Smith, MS, RN, CNAA, BC
M. Janice Nelson, EdD, RN
Angela Barron McBride, PhD, RN, FAAN
G. Rumay Alexander, EdD, RN

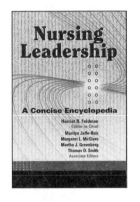

"We are delighted to introduce this book to a new generation of readers. The challenges in nursing, as well as in health care, have never been greater. The need for resources such as this text is profound."

—From the Foreword by **Joanne Disch**, PhD, RN, FAAN,
School of Nursing, University of Minnesota
and **Kathleen Dracup**, DNSc, FNP, RN, FAAN,
School of Nursing, University of California, San Francisco

Nursing Leadership: A Concise Encyclopedia is a manageable, one-volume reference that describes and defines the field of nursing leadership. The *Encyclopedia* will provide students, faculty, nurse managers, executives, and others with a comprehensive resource for information about the range of knowledge and roles encompassed by the term "nursing leadership." It details the contributions of key nursing leaders, the knowledge base and traits of leadership, skills and models on which leadership is based, the regulatory environment of health care, the range of practice settings and roles, and the design of quality outcomes.

The editors and contributors to this essential reference comprise some of the best-known and influential leaders in the nursing field. This book will be a cherished resource for leaders and future leaders in health care.

2008 · 608 pp · Hardcover · 978-0-8261-0258-4

11 West 42nd Street, New York, NY 10036-8002 • Fax: 212-941-7842
Order Toll-Free: 877-687-7476 • Order Online: www.springerpub.com

Leadership and Management Skills for Long-Term Care

Eileen M. Sullivan-Marx, PhD, RNC, FAAN
Deanna Gray-Miceli, DNSc, APRN, Editors

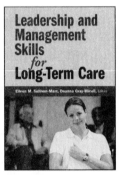

While the scope of long-term-care settings has expanded from nursing homes and home care agencies to assisted living facilities and community-based health services, the training for nurses, managers and administrators, medical directors, and other professionals who work in these facilities is often fragmented. This book was developed to fill a widely recognized gap in the management and leadership skills of RNs needed to improve the quality of long-term care. The book is based around learning modules in leadership and management competencies that were site-tested in three types of long-term-care settings and revised based on the resulting feedback. Several of the nurse experts involved in the project contribute to this book.

The leadership modules cover team building, communication, power and negotiation, change theory and process, management direction and design, and management that moves from conflict to collaboration. Two additional modules cover cultural competence and principles of teaching and learning related to adult education in the long-term-care environment. Together, these skills will enhance the nurse's ability to build and interact with the geriatric care team, resolve conflict, negotiate for solutions, develop collaboration, and teach and mentor nurses and nursing assistants.

Key Features of this book:

- Addresses the gap in RN preparation in leadership and management skills in long-term-care settings
- Easy-to-use modules suitable for self-learning or group training
- Modules include pre- and post-tests, learning objectives, case studies, and materials for hand-outs

2008 · 200 pp · Hardcover · 978-0-8261-5993-9

11 West 42nd Street, New York, NY 10036-8002 • Fax: 212-941-7842
Order Toll-Free: 877-687-7476 • Order Online: www.springerpub.com